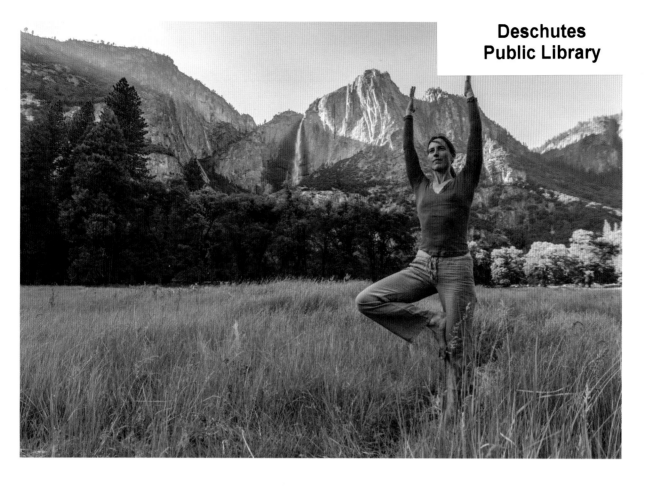

THE OUTDOOR ADVENTURER'S
GUIDE TO YOGA

Practices for Strong and Balanced Hiking, Climbing, Paddling, and Cycling

JANA KILGORE
Photographs by Patrick Brems

FALCONGUIDES

GUILFORD, CONNECTICUT

FALCONGUIDES®

An imprint of Globe Pequot, the trade division of
The Rowman & Littlefield Publishing Group, Inc.
4501 Forbes Blvd., Ste. 200
Lanham, MD 20706
Falcon.com
Falcon and FalconGuides are registered trademarks and Make Adventure Your Story is a
trademark of The Rowman & Littlefield Publishing Group, Inc.

Distributed by NATIONAL BOOK NETWORK

British Library Cataloguing in Publication Information available

Library of Congress Cataloging-in-Publication Data

Names: Kilgore, Jana, 1976– author.
Title: The outdoor adventurer's guide to yoga : practices for strong and balanced hiking,
    climbing, paddling, and cycling / Jana Kilgore ; photographs by Patrick Bremser.
Description: Guilford, Connecticut : Falcon, [2021] | Includes bibliographical references
    and index. | Summary: "Guide to the foundations of yoga, anatomy, alignment, breath
    work, and asana that applies these practices specifically for hiking, backpacking, cycling,
    climbing, paddling, and snow sports"— Provided by publisher.
Identifiers: LCCN 2021011876 (print) | LCCN 2021011877 (ebook) | ISBN
    9781493055289 (paperback) | ISBN 9781493055296 (epub)
Subjects: LCSH: Hatha yoga—Popular works. | Outdoor recreation.
Classification: LCC RA781.7 .K49 2021 (print) | LCC RA781.7 (ebook) | DDC
    613.7/046--dc23
LC record available at https://lccn.loc.gov/2021011876
LC ebook record available at https://lccn.loc.gov/2021011877

♾™ The paper used in this publication meets the minimum requirements of American
National Standard for Information Sciences—Permanence of Paper for Printed Library
Materials, ANSI/NISO Z39.48-1992.

CONTENTS

ACKNOWLEDGMENTS   v

FOREWORD   vii

INTRODUCTION   ix

1   Foundations of Yoga   1

2   Anatomy Basics   15

3   Alignment Principles   27

4   Yoga of Breathing   41

5   *Asana*   47

6   Yoga for Hiking   143

7   Yoga for Backpacking   167

8   Yoga for Paddling   181

9   Yoga for Cycling   195

10   Yoga for Climbing   213

11   Yoga for Snow Sports   227

12   Building a Home Practice   241

13   Yoga for Recovering   253

REFERENCES   266

RESOURCES   268

INDEX   270

ABOUT THE AUTHOR   275

ABOUT THE CONTRIBUTORS   276

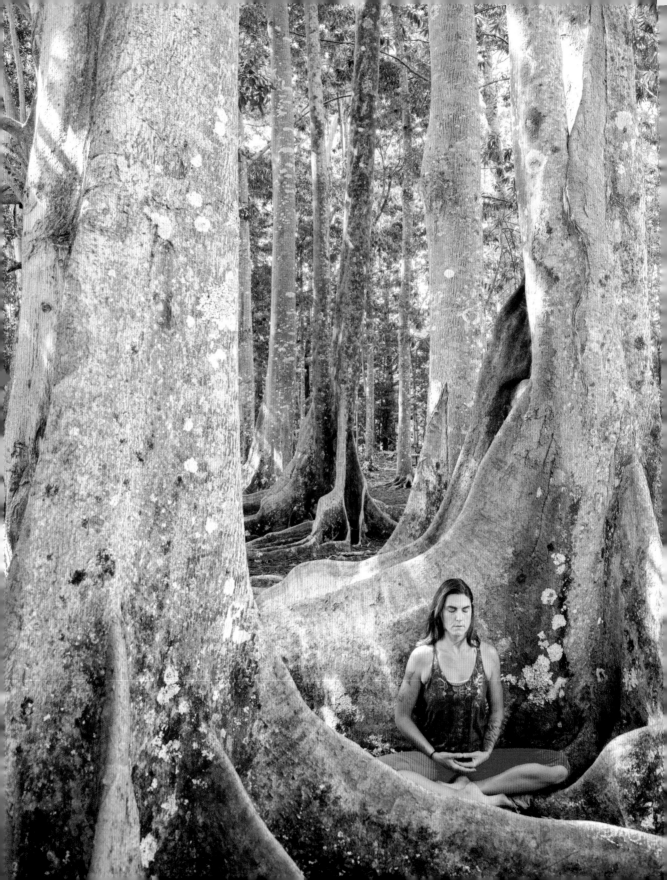

ACKNOWLEDGMENTS

SO MANY INCREDIBLE PEOPLE HELPED MAKE THIS BOOK POSSIBLE; I will do my best to acknowledge them all. My early influences were mainly Mother Nature herself, my supportive, loving parents, and my brothers who were surfing, skating, and playing hard at everything they could, always inspiring me to get outside. While I did not have the chance to meet them in person, Ram Dass and Gurumayi Chidvilasanada's teachings on meditation and life have shaped my path. Many yoga and Ayurveda teachers have passed on their wisdom and experience, backed by generations of teachers before them. Among the most influential to my yoga and Ayurveda practice and teaching are Theresa Elliott, Desiree Rumbaugh, Noah Maze, Jennifer Prugh, Douglas Brooks, Sonam Targee, Dr. Robert Svaboda, and Dr. Scott Blossom. To my soul sisters at Balanced Rock Foundation, Heather Sullivan and Eliza Kerr, I give deep thanks for their invitation to learn guiding and join them in leading people into the magic of Yosemite National Park. Thanks to my amazing editor, Katherine O'Dell, and the incredible team at FalconGuides for putting this book together and holding my hand along the way. To the many new and old friends I interviewed for the book, you constantly inspire me, thank you. To my students, clients, and retreat participants over the years, thank you for teaching me so much and sharing your joys and struggles with me. I especially want to acknowledge and thank my supportive, loving, and incredibly talented husband, Patrick Bremser, who always has my back. He took most of the beautiful photos in the book and made outdoor yoga photo shoots fun for everyone. To my friends who modeled for the asana section, Tulasi Adeva Perrin, Monica Chung, Candice Neeves, Nathan Myers, Sarah Kortschak, and Jacob Dinger, thank you for supporting this project and for demonstrating such strength and grace. A special note of thanks to Quinn Brett for her suggestions on adaptive yoga and adventure, yoga, and sustainable living in harmony with nature. May this book be a source of inspiration, healing, and strength for your adventures ahead.

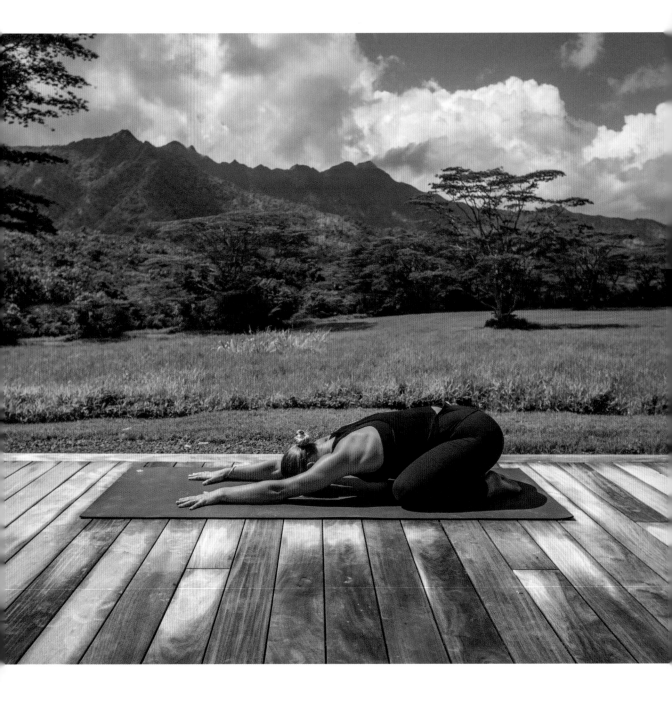

FOREWORD

WE ARE ALL ATHLETES, JUGGLING CHILDREN, JOBS, JOYS, and passions. I was a professional athlete, a climber, a mountain runner, and a triathlete. Yoga has been a part of my life, my routine, since gymnastics fell away from my heart in high school. Athletics was a shining platform to explore myself, mentally and physically. Yoga deepened my experience and exploration. How can I adapt a muscle or the mind to find comfort in the uncomfortable?

In 2017, I took a life-altering climbing fall. I broke my back and sustained a spinal cord injury. The legs, glutes, and core that I so playfully explored the mountains and the mat with were left paralyzed, motionless. Early in my recovery discomfort was overwhelming. I had a new body that wasn't participating and a mind that was wandering, wishing, blaming, and unfocused. I felt defeated and hopeless. Joy was so far away.

Maybe half a year into this new existence, I found myself on the floor. Exploring the space on my yoga mat. Exploring the vulnerable space in my mind. Exploring the small firings of muscles and a playful awkwardness of balance poses. I found that my yoga practice was still available to me. Patience and exploration were mandatory . . . the same as it was prior to my injury.

Jana's encounters exploring the wild places of our natural world transfer to her understanding of yoga and the wild spaces of our minds. She clearly conveys the importance of incorporating a simple breath of fresh air and a vast landscape to better manage the unexpected milieu life throws at us. We need to care for ourselves, just as we need to care for the natural landscape that surrounds us. We need to balance taking and giving.

While I am still looking for peace with my new body, I am lucky to have teachers like Jana to remind me of both the mental and the physical progress. Reminding us that beauty and calm is always available to us, especially when we need it most, as we endeavor into our sports.

The Outdoor Adventurer's Guide to Yoga is adaptive to all of us as we evolve our practice on this ever-evolving planet, at any time on our spectrum and life and capability. Whether you are an elite athlete or dabbling with expanding your sphere of exploration, Jana and this fantastic resource will guide you through.

—Quinn Brett
Director of Accessibility, National Park Service
Yogi, writer, athlete

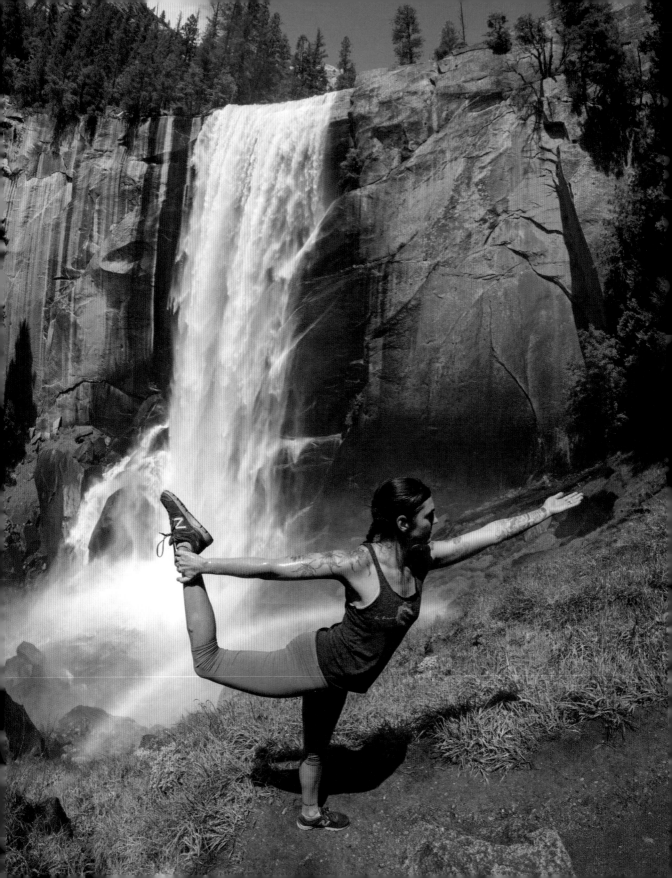

INTRODUCTION

THIS BOOK WAS BORN IN A MOMENT OF AWE for the power of yoga in the wild. I was fresh off the trail from leading a yoga and backpacking trip in Yosemite National Park. We'd headed off into the backcountry and basked in the glory of the wilderness, soaking in the power of the practices. Fields of wildflowers, cold alpine lakes, happy, tired hiking companions, and starry skies had filled our days and nights. My head was swimming with the feedback from our participants and from the incredible experiences of the last week at high altitude when this opportunity arose. In reflecting on that humbling moment, a chance to share this practice with so many outdoor enthusiasts, I looked back at what my life would have been without yoga. If it were not for my practice of yoga over the years, these outdoor experiences would have remained out of reach. Without the strength, flexibility, focus, and equanimity my practice provides, I would not be able to get out there—off-road, off-trail—out in the wild. I think everyone can benefit from learning and practicing the art and science of yoga. There is a saying that as long as you can breathe you can practice yoga. Every day I am thankful for that breath and all the ways yoga makes my life better—on the mat, on the trail, and in life.

Yoga has long supported my outdoor adventures. I prepare and recover from backpacking and hiking with yoga. My daily practice helps keep my body, mind, and breath balanced. Taking time during a hike to stop, release tight muscles, slow my breath and body down, and enjoy my surroundings helps me be more present for the experience and awakens my senses to take it all in. Honestly, I don't know how I could thru-hike without a recovery practice each day, or a pre-hike practice each morning. All these years, miles, and down dogs have shown me that life, and hiking, is better with yoga. My hope is that this guide provides the tools, information, and inspiration for outdoor athletes and enthusiasts to develop a yoga practice that helps them enjoy more days outdoors adventuring for many years to come.

When I was younger my approach to yoga was much more athletic, focused on achieving challenging poses and practices. But the more time I spend outside pursuing sports, the less the outer shape of a pose matters and the more the inner awareness and experience does. My approach now is to cultivate balance, steadiness, strength, mobility, and sustainability in my practice and life. Learning new sports and trying new adventures demands more of me and shows me both where I am strong

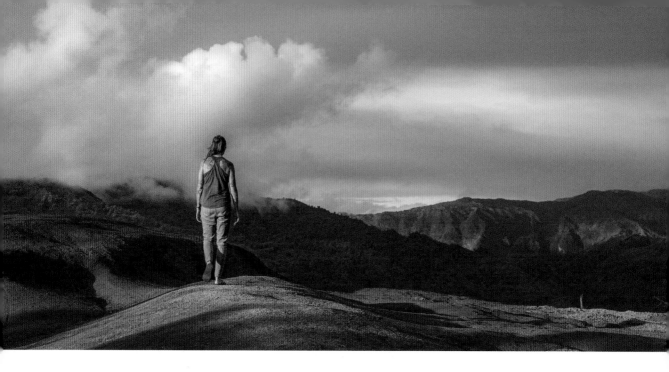

and where I am compromised. My yoga practice is a place where I can work, daily, with imbalances and become more whole and aware. Key to the power of yoga, though, is practicing each of the eight limbs of *Hatha* yoga, both on and off the mat. This is not just a book on *asanas* and stretching, but one integrating a yogic life with an outdoor enthusiast and steward's life. Really, the same principles apply.

I will share my experiences of practicing yoga and different sequences for different sports, as well as insights from experts in the field of yoga, alignment, functional movement, meditation, and self-care. Athletes from a range of outdoor sports will also share their experiences of practicing yoga and its benefits in their lives. I hope that everyone, from beginners to experienced practitioners, can be inspired and benefit from this book.

How to Use This Book

The beginning of this book outlines a foundation for practicing yoga skillfully. Having a firm understanding of the philosophy and framework of yoga guides us in safely and effectively weaving yoga practices into our lives. The anatomy chapter lays the groundwork for understanding the body, especially the musculoskeletal system, and aids in a common language for understanding the instructions for breathing and posture. The *asana* chapter covers all the postures that are in the sport-specific sequences located in each sport's chapter. Each posture and practice includes the benefits of the posture, instructions for getting into and out of the postures, as well as adaptations and notes on safety.

With this foundation in yoga, you can go to the chapters that cover your individual sports and begin practicing the sequences for training, warming up, and recovering from your adventure. If you engage in multiple sports, get familiar with the demands of each sport and begin practicing the sequences for each one. Most likely your sports vary with the seasons, so practice the sequences for snow sports fall through spring and the paddling or backpacking sequences spring through fall, for instance. There is also a general yoga sequence that benefits athletes of any sport. Use this anytime as a daily practice.

The chapter on recovery practices benefits all, and I encourage you to read it through and pick at least one type of practice to begin working with based on what calls to you. If you are recovering from an injury or illness, the restorative yoga and meditation practices are extremely helpful in the healing process. If you are training for a competition or adventure, incorporating *yoga nidra* into your weekly practice benefits the nervous system and strengthens neural pathways for better performance and a positive mindset.

Remember that yoga is a practice, a way of living in close connection with our own nature and the rhythms of nature itself. Start where you are and begin to explore the practices, letting them develop over time.

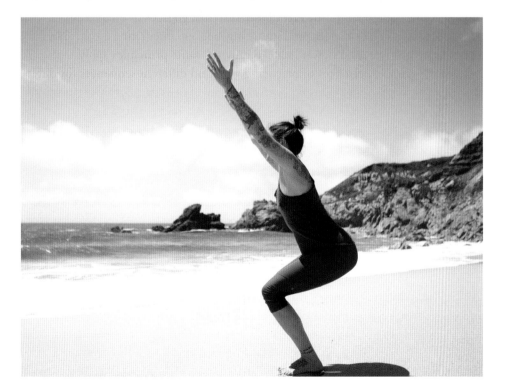

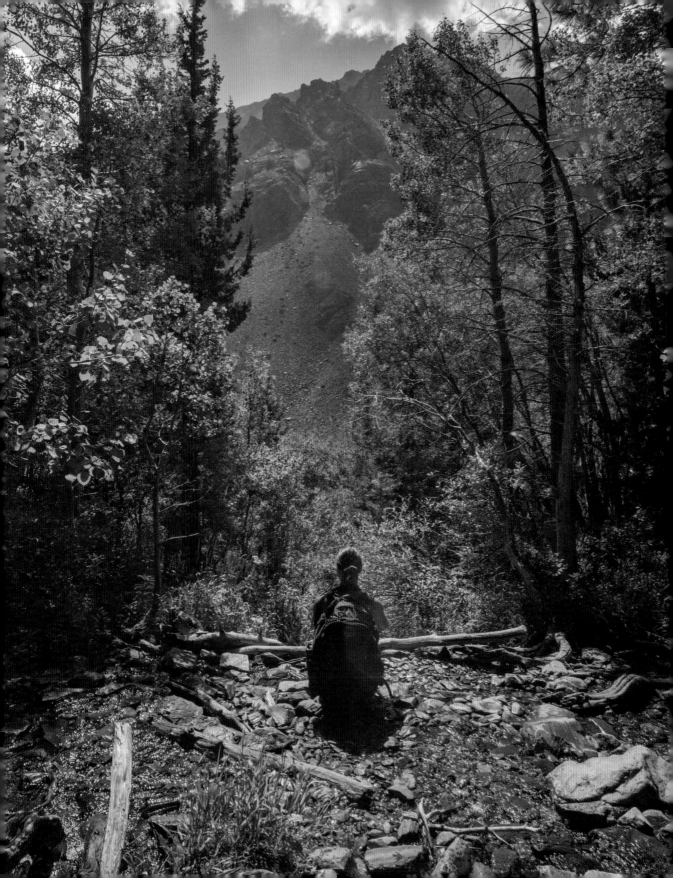

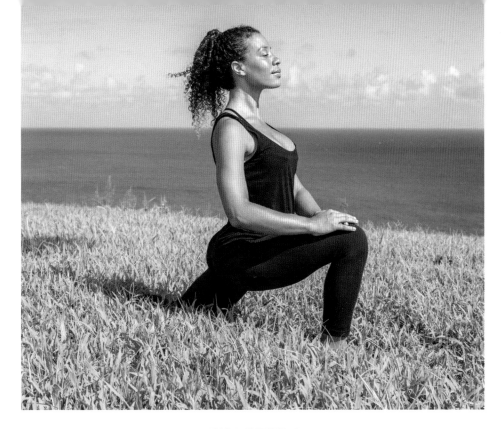

CHAPTER 1

FOUNDATIONS OF YOGA

The very heart of yoga practice is "abyhasa" steady
effort in the direction you want to go.
—SALLY KEMPTON

YOGA, MEANING "TO YOKE," "TO JOIN," OR "UNION," is the ancient system
of holistic and harmonious living that arose from diverse and evolving cultures
on the Indian subcontinent. While it is influenced by various traditions, including
Hindu, Buddhist, and Jain, the philosophy, teaching, and practice of yoga are vast
and beyond any religion. It is an ancient science of positive transformation that is
applicable to anyone, anywhere in time. Slowly, the practice changes our patterns on
a physical, mental, and emotional level to create inner and outer alignment.

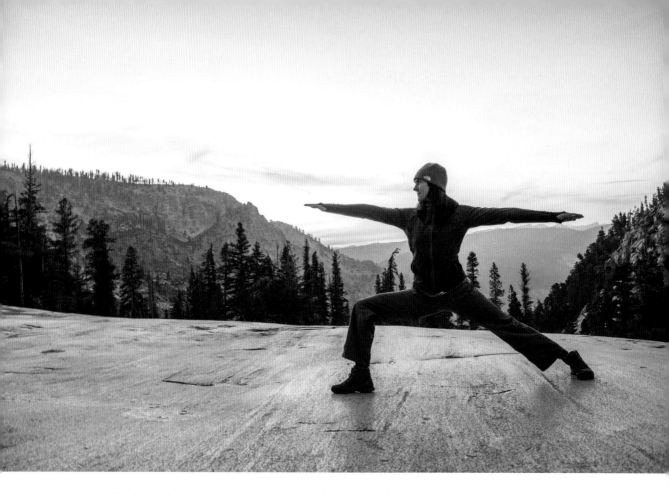

Traditionally yoga was passed from student to teacher via oral and physical teaching as well as through ancient texts, songs, and practices. Nowadays there are many lineages—different styles for different people and different times of life. What we think of as yoga in modern times is mostly the postures, called *asanas*, yet this is only one aspect of the yoga tradition that is *Hatha* yoga, the practice of disciplines that lead to evolution on every level. One of the older yogic texts, the *Yoga Sutras* by the sage Patanjali, explains eight limbs or types of practice for an engaged, balanced, and healthy life.

> TIED TO THE IDEA OF TAKING AN ACTIVE SEAT WITHIN THE BODY AND MIND, AS OPPOSED TO OUR NORMAL DISTRACTION FROM THE BODY BY THE BUSY MIND, IS TO PRACTICE POSTURES WITH STEADINESS (*STHIRA*) AND SOFTNESS (*SUKHA*)."

EIGHT LIMBS OF YOGA

Yamas

The first are the *yamas*, the principles of ethical behavior for our relationships with ourselves and others. Meaning "to control" or "to contain," the *yamas* help us navigate life's ups and downs with grace. These five principles build a foundation that encompasses all of life at home and on outdoor adventures.

Ahimsa: Often translated as "non-harming," "non-violence," or "active kindness," it begins with practicing kindness and non-harming toward ourselves and extends to all other beings in the world. *Ahimsa* in the outdoors means opening our eyes to the effects of our presence and activities. It guides us to leave a place as we found it, and to not harm animals and environments.

Satya: This is the principle of honesty, truthfulness, and actively not deceiving ourselves or others. *Ahimsa* informs *satya*, so when practicing honesty, always ask yourself if what you are about to say is kind, true, and necessary. This can come into play when interacting with others in the outdoors. *Satya* inspires us to ask, how can we best communicate for the good of the whole?

Asteya: Translated as "not stealing," this is in essence the practice of releasing desire for what we do not have or haven't earned through honest work and means. This includes not taking what is not ours without permission. It means following park regulations and often leaving behind a beautiful stone, pinecone, or leaf. It challenges the notion that something is ours simply because we found it or want it.

Brahmacharya: Traditionally this word is translated as "celibacy," directing ancient yogis to focus solely on the path of enlightenment, harnessing their energy. Modern interpretations of this principle speak to respect and integrity in relationships, especially intimate ones, and honoring our own personal energy as well as others. This might mean resisting every urge we have to run off-trail, achieve the highest peak even if we're pushing daylight, or otherwise put our physical desires ahead of all else.

Aparigraha: Similar to *asteya* this principle means "non-covetousness" or "non-hoarding." Living simply, with a content and generous heart, means we are not being greedy or taking more than what we need. On a personal scale it is sharing water and food with your fellow adventurers. Practicing *aparigraha* might even help you keep your pack light, challenging your need for every possession you might want on the trail.

Niyamas

The second limb of yoga turns from the external to the internal. The *niyamas* are the personal guidelines for a healthy relationship with ourselves on a physical, mental, and emotional level. Following these guiding principles enhances our personal health and well-being as we take responsibility for ourselves.

Saucha: Often translated as "cleanliness" or "purity," this principle is one of tending to the physical body to support proper elimination and detoxification. Bathing regularly, oral hygiene, hydration, a balanced diet, and elimination are all recommended. When the body is functioning properly, we can enjoy our time in nature and with others. Since physical health and mental/emotional health are interconnected, tending to the body aids in mental clarity and calm.

Santosha: The *yamas* and *saucha* make it possible for the mind, body, and heart to become "content," the common translation of this principle. It is meeting life on life's terms, practicing self-acceptance and enjoying the journey. This helps us be present in our outdoor activities, and in the capacity of our body as well. In practice it is being happy with what we can do now and helps dissolve the desire to be someone or something else than we are right now.

Tapas: This Sanskrit word means "to be hot" and refers to the heat created by friction, rubbing, or steady pressure that is sustained over a period of time—like the repetition and dedication that creates strength, stamina, and skill. It's the effort to train for a sport, a race, or a big adventure. Discipline, steady focus on a goal, and the right effort help us become better humans. Steady pressure in a positive direction also helps us prepare for a trip or training session, giving it our best and relaxing afterward. You'll notice the literal heat that builds during this work. In the context of yoga, that heat does more than make you sweat.

Svadhyaya: "Self-study" and "self-reflection" are some translations of this word. It includes contemplation practices and the study of spiritual texts and sacred works. We intentionally practice self-awareness in all we do in the world, reflect regularly for inner guidance, and know when we need to change course. On a trail, river, boulder, or slope, self-reflection tells us how we need to prepare, if we are prepared, and how we are really doing along the way.

Ishvarapranidhana: This may be one of the most challenging principles for many people. "Surrendering to a higher power or God" looks different for everyone. The idea is to open to what is bigger than us, to life energy itself, to nature, the cosmos, the unknown. It is a way of taking our place among the infinite and remembering we are part of a whole that is carrying us at all times. In nature we can experience this spontaneously at the top of a mountain, skiing fresh powder with spectacular views, or paddling at sunset. We experience the magnificence of this power greater than ourselves in these moments of connection.

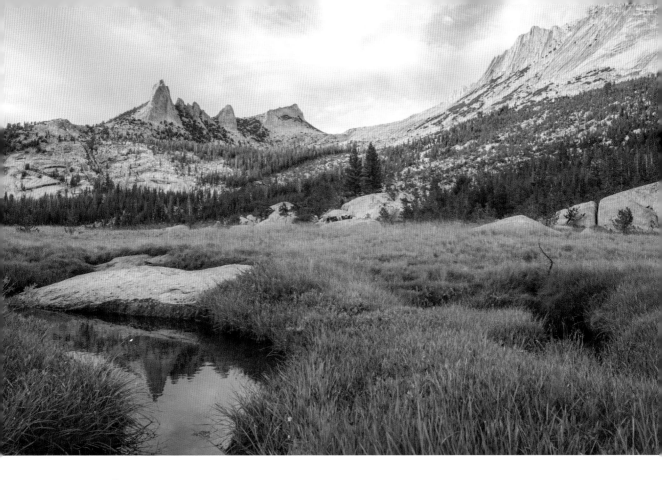

Asana

While the *Yoga Sutras* do not discuss any postural practices specifically, they do describe the way and the goal of practice. The root of the word *asana* is the idea of inhabiting, existing, and living with presence in our body. It refers to firmly establishing ourselves within the body and the ritual practice of doing so. This requires dedication and physical stability, as well as attention and mental discipline. All the movement and exertion of physical yoga isn't just to condition the body for peak performance, but to allow the mind to be still.

Tied to the idea of taking an active seat within the body and mind, as opposed to our normal distraction from the body by the busy mind, is to practice postures with steadiness (*sthira*) and softness (*sukha*). As we move from pose to pose on and off the mat, we do so with strength and ease, without excessive force both in body and mind. In this way we develop a state of equilibrium also known as *sattva* in Sanskrit. Of course, this takes practice. When we are learning to climb or ski, we are clumsy at first, and our movements can feel clunky instead of graceful. With patience and persistence we find the flow and ease within our sports and activities that lead to that essential state of awareness and joy.

Pranayama

The next limb of yoga according to the *Yoga Sutras* is *pranayama*, controlling the inhalation and exhalation with a steady and easeful posture. Classically this limb is introduced after one has a steady physical practice of *asana*. Once the body and mind have become more established, balanced, and calm, then working with breathing practices can be done with greater ease and benefit. There are many different breath practices; the most basic one, *ujayii*, will be explained in Chapter 4: Yoga of Breathing (page 41). Expanding our breath capacity helps increase our energy levels and keeps the mind clear and focused for greater endurance. Some of the breathing techniques in chapter 4 help to regulate the nervous system and keep us calm during challenging experiences, helpful in all realms of life and especially in the wild.

Pratyahara

The practice of withdrawing the senses inward, taking a break from all the external stimuli around us, is the next limb of yoga. Since the mind tends to either grasp or push away from stimulation, it is always wandering. By drawing the senses inward and training our minds to occasionally withdraw, we not only calm and nurture the senses but also bring the mind into a more peaceful state. This allows the physiology of the body to function more optimally and keeps our senses attuned to both our inner and outer environment. In my opinion, literally withdrawing from civilization and getting out into nature is one of the most effective ways of practicing *pratyahara*. It is also useful for increasing our ability to concentrate, which leads us to the next limb.

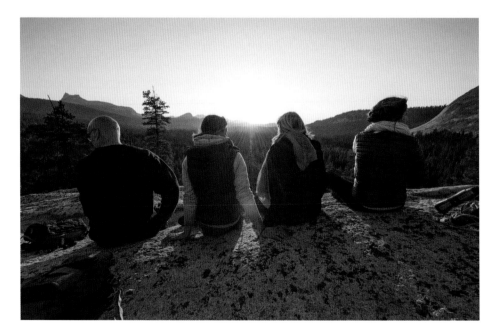

Dharana

When we have developed a stronger connection to our senses, using them wisely, resting them, and nurturing them through *pratyahara*, our ability to focus the mind on one point increases. We experience less distraction from the world around us and develop sustained concentration. This is the essence of *dharana*. Much of the time when people are meditating, they are practicing keeping their attention on one thing. The mind wanders often, as is its nature, and we gently bring it back to the point of focus. Perhaps we are focusing on our breath, our body, a word, an image, or thoughts passing by—much like lying on a warm slab of granite in the mountains and watching the sky. Clouds and birds pass by, and we notice them, but our attention remains on the sky itself. This is one of many concentration practices that help build mental, emotional, and physical stamina.

Dhyana

As we progress through the limbs, we can see how they build upon each other. Just as hiking builds into backpacking, which leads to ever more remote and epic destinations, and as skateboarding might lead to surfing and snowboarding—practices are progressive. The skills developed lead to all kinds of new possibilities and greater depth of experience. Once we have developed the ability to concentrate for long periods, we can become absorbed into the experience of oneness. This is the goal of meditation, *dhyana*.

Dharana cultivates intermittent moments of focused attention. When the attention becomes sustained and steady, it leads us to *dhyana* or meditation. At first these moments of attention are fleeting. But just as individual raindrops in a constant storm become streams carving into the earth, this focused attention helps us dig into states of meditation.

Samadhi

The eighth and final limb of yoga is *samadhi*, enlightenment. While there are the rare few individuals who have attained a state of transcendence or enlightenment, it is not just for sages and monks living a hermetic life on the mountain. A more modern interpretation is to be in a state of sustained and intense presence and objectivity. In essence, you perceive all points of view of reality at once, taking all into consideration in your observance.

Many modern meditation teachers describe enlightenment as complete absorption in reality as it is, without judgment. It is a state we may experience at different times of our lives and seek again and again. As outdoor athletes you may have experienced something like this during a once-in-a-lifetime climb, a peak moment during a backpacking trip, during a sublime sunrise paddle, or on a night under the

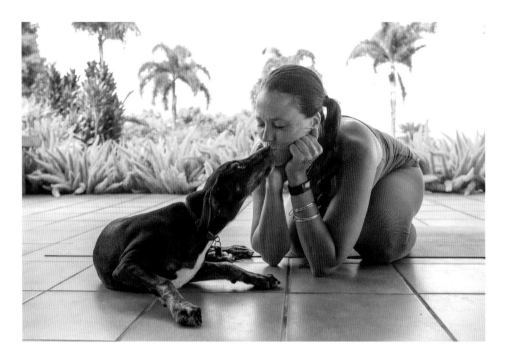

aurora borealis after a day on the slopes. I think it is our very nature as humans and outdoor adventurers to seek this state and connection with the vastness of the cosmos, the power all around and within.

BENEFITS OF YOGA

So what are the benefits of yoga for outdoor athletes? Well, the same as for all humans really. Yoga helps build and balance muscle strength and improve posture as we age. It helps improve mobility and increase range of motion. This, of course, varies widely among people due to the great diversity in skeletal structure as well as physiological differences. Balance is improved both in motion as well as in static holds, which greatly reduces the risk of falling and subsequent injuries. Yoga also improves physical and mental agility by improving reaction time.

The physical practice helps improve coordination and endurance, as well as increase bone density. Building the core muscles of the torso that support the spine reduces the risk of joint injury. This also helps us move with more grace, strength, and longevity. Building a balanced body brings various muscle groups in sync, meaning each movement and engagement works together, reducing individual muscle fatigue.

Pranayama, the breathing practices of yoga, help us expand lung capacity, regulate our breathing, and keep us more calm and alert. We can use breath awareness as a self-check-in to see how we are doing and if we might need to take some deeper breaths or even rest a bit. With regular practice we can recover faster as well.

The mental discipline and incorporating the personal and social principles in the *yamas* and *niyamas* also help us make wiser choices in training, stretching, recovery, and navigating challenges out in nature. When we are facing the last mile climb of an extreme elevation hike with 40 pounds on our backs, we can choose to go at a safe pace, rest more often, use hiking poles, and develop the mental toughness and gratitude that will get us safely to the top. These principles also encourage us to keep an eye on our companions along the way, helping out where we can.

Yoga teaches us mindfulness, which is the practice of focusing our minds and bodies in each moment to be fully present. We engage our whole selves—mind, body, heart, and senses—in what we are doing and experiencing. Mindfulness can be practiced on the mat, trail, slope, river, or big wall, as well as when setting up camp, washing the dishes, and folding laundry. It is the act of bringing ourselves back to the moment again and again with full awareness.

Meditation and yoga can help improve neuroplasticity, the ability of the brain to actually create new neural pathways and habits. This improves mental functioning, resiliency, and problem solving. Relaxation practices such as *yoga nidra*, also known as yogic sleep, can shift the brain waves from gamma, the fully awake state, to alpha and theta, the conscious and subconscious levels of thinking. A weekly yogic sleep practice of just 20 to 30 minutes has shown evidence of improving stress response, decreasing muscle tension, and improving overall sense of well-being. A daily meditation practice of 20 to 30 minutes has been shown to help with stress management, sleep, anxiety and depression, anger, and self-compassion. A 2018 study showed that *asana* and meditation practices reduce the amygdala volume on the right side of the brain. This is the area that is associated with negative emotions and the fear response. There are more studies happening all the time that help validate the experience and wisdom of this ancient system of yoga. It doesn't matter if you sit on a cushion in lotus pose, on a chair with your feet grounded, or even in a kayak. Meditation and mindfulness practices work when we start where we are, do the best we can, and practice consistently, just like any new sport we try.

For the purposes of this book, this is as far as we will go into the foundations of yoga and its philosophy. At its roots this is a way of life, just like being an environmentally conscious adventurer. This is a holistic way of engaging with ourselves and the world around us. The guiding principles of the *yamas* and *niyamas* can deepen our inner and outer well-being and help us be more loving and nurturing as we navigate the changes of life and our evolution as human beings engaging with the natural world. Leading with *ahimsa*, non-harming, we approach the practices of yoga in a way that helps us be more balanced, wise, and compassionate with ourselves and others as we engage in the activities that bring us so much joy. The Leave No Trace principles weave the yogic principles into how we steward our natural world as well.

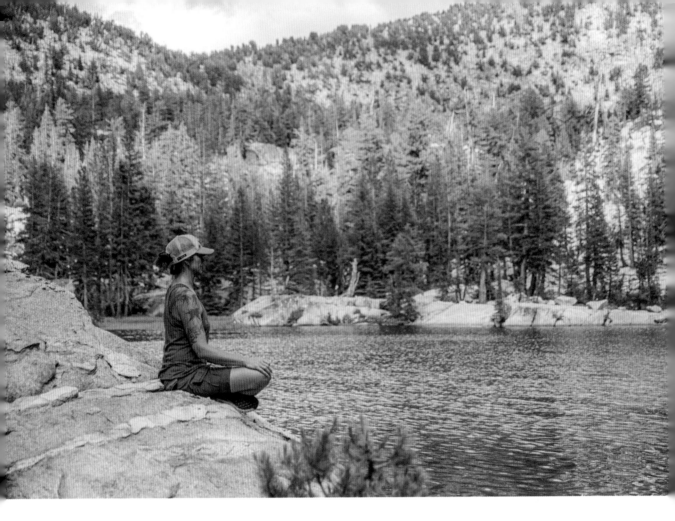

Leave No Trace

- **Plan ahead and prepare:** This leads to wise action and helps us navigate challenges we may face on adventures. Practicing yoga to prepare the body and mind, choosing the best time to take a paddle or hike, and practicing kindness and honesty along the journey are some ways to bring this principle to life.

- **Travel and camp on durable surfaces:** This is non-harming in action. It reduces impact on the environment and risk as we travel.

- **Dispose of waste properly:** By respecting our natural environment and packing our waste out, we reduce harm and practice honesty.

- **Leave what you find:** By not taking what does not belong to us, we reduce our "stealing," practice honesty, and practice reducing our desires. Observe the beauty, take a picture, and leave the plant, rock, or pinecone.

YOGI INSIGHT

JENNIFER PRUGH
founder of Breathe Together Yoga and Joy of Yoga 200-
300 Hour Training, photographer and author; CA.

How do you use the *yamas* and *niyamas* in daily life?
When I learned about them, they provided a template for living my life. I liked guidelines, not rules. It meant I could work with them at my own pace and in my own way. I was fascinated with all of them but then learned that if I could remember just two (non-violence and truth), they would encompass all of them. The *yamas* are about working with others, the *niyamas* with one's self. But I use them interchangeably with self and others. The way I use them now is if I'm suffering in any way I pause to look at which *yama* or *niyama* needs my attention. I ask myself, "What is the nature of the suffering? Is it attachment, ego, untruth, envy?"

I view the *yamas* and *niyamas* much like remedies. There are periods where there are themes in life that come up. Such as with Covid. There is a *niyama* about finding some contentment in the midst of real difficulty. Even if I am struggling with a given situation, and there have been many hard situations, I can say to myself, "I can be here in this moment. I can do this." It's a one-step-at-a-time approach that involves a great deal less "fight or flight."

How has your relationship with the eight limbs changed over time?
My interpretation of each limb has changed over the years. Rather than trying to "get somewhere" with *asana*, my focus now is on "being here." I also really appreciate and am experimenting with the idea that the *asana* practice is about developing real love. As a hard-driving practitioner for a number of years, this has been revelatory. I use the *yamas* and *niyamas* to enter meditation as well. It helps me focus and navigate through layers of thought very effectively.

How can outdoor athletes connect with the eight limbs of yoga?
These principles are time tested, and they basically help us be better people to ourselves and others. The eight limbs guide us in navigating through life, to the extent to which we wish to be guided. What are the ethics that we will stand for? When we lie to ourselves, how does that go for us? What is the code that we live by? I think that the eight limbs can support every aspect of our lives and help us actively respect the life we have been given, and life in general.

What's the biggest point you think people should focus on in the outdoors and indoors?
Presence. Get present in every area of your life, anywhere you are. Life is amazing! There is always something to totally appreciate.

Mindfulness, meditation, *asana*, and breathwork are the practice of being in the now. Everything good happens in the present moment, not the past or future.

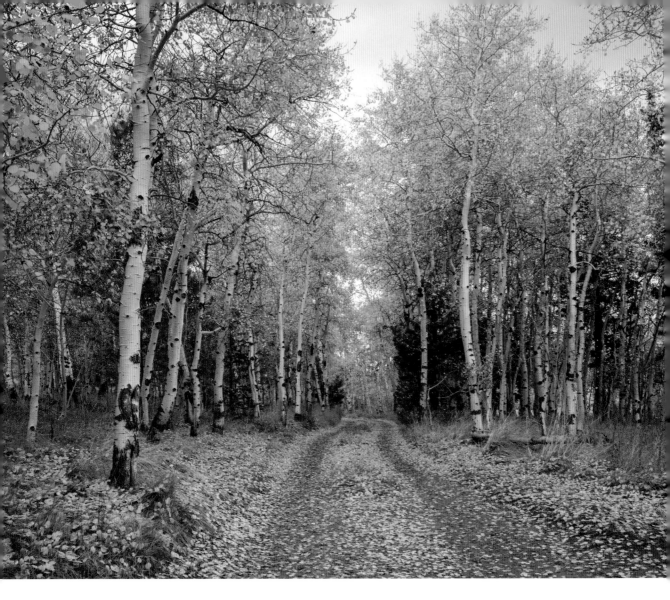

- **Minimize campfire effects:** Another act of non-harming is choosing when and where to have a campfire, minimizing any damaging effects of fire on the environment we are enjoying and caring for.

- **Respect wildlife:** When we adventure in the wild, we are in someone else's home. Respecting wildlife is practicing kindness, respect, and safety for all.

- **Be considerate of other visitors:** Be kind and gracious to others who are out seeking adventure and playing in nature as well. We each have a responsibility to care for nature and to work together to reduce pollution and impact of all kinds.

THE TAKEAWAY

Yoga, an ancient science and method of deep transformation on all levels, is a holistic way of living in harmony with nature, each other, and ourselves. One of my teachers says that yoga helps us be better humans and better at whatever our vocation is. It helps us show up for life as it truly is, and love and accept ourselves as we are throughout our personal evolution. No matter the sport it can help us be more fully present, physically and mentally capable, and more connected to the world around us.

- The eight limbs of yoga are a framework for living a more intentional life, beginning with how we treat ourselves and how we interact with others and the world.

- Practicing postures and breathing with compassion and honesty helps us be more attuned to our physical patterns of movement and can help repattern our nervous systems to be more calm and centered.

- Training our minds to focus and stay present helps us to not only achieve states of oneness such as meditation but also be mindful in our outdoor activities through challenge and triumph.

- Practicing yoga can help us bring greater balance, strength, and courage to our adventures and training while also reducing injury and risk.

- There is a beautiful synergy between the *yamas* and *niyamas* and the Leave No Trace principles, helping us be better stewards of the natural world that brings us so much joy.

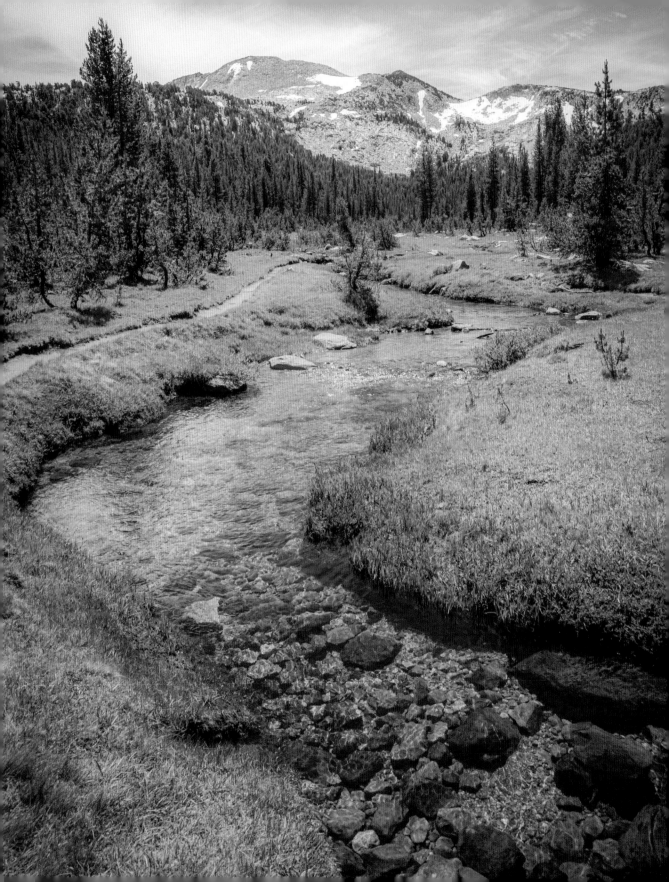

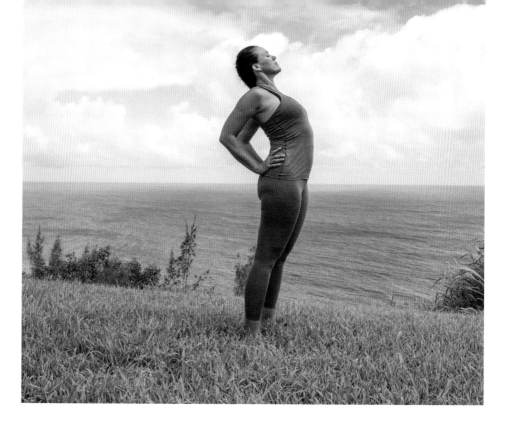

CHAPTER 2

ANATOMY BASICS

To keep the body in good health is a duty . . . otherwise we
shall not be able to keep our mind strong and clear.
—BUDDHA

WHOLE BODY CONNECTION

The individual postures of yoga are based on a cohesive understanding of the whole
body. Yoga affects the entire body and all of its systems. Practices are based on an
ancient belief in the interconnectedness of the body that Western science is beginning to catch up with. Our mental state affects our nervous system; our breathing,
circulation, digestion, and endocrine system; and every other system of the body. Yoga
philosophy views the whole body as a dynamic and complex system—everything
affecting everything else—and aims to create integration. Modern research shows

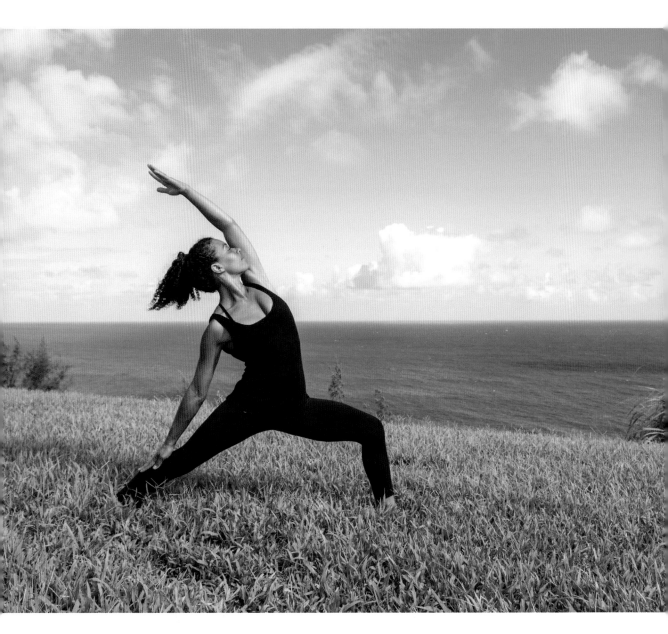

that our thoughts affect the functioning of each cell. This is part of why the mind-body practice of yoga has wide-ranging benefits, helping create optimal functioning on every level. For the purposes of this book and beginning or deepening your practice of yoga to support your outdoor lifestyle, we will cover the basic anatomy of the body to aid in understanding the importance of alignment, functional movement, and sustainable health.

STRUCTURE

The entire musculoskeletal system is composed of muscle, bone, and connective tissue. The body's 206 bones are made of collagen and store calcium. Bones create the structure and stability of the body, muscles attach to bones via tendons, and bones attach to other bones by ligaments. Joints are a complex matrix of ligaments, tendons, cartilage, and fluids where two bones meet. Muscles move the skeleton and insulate the body. While muscles have a high amount of elastin that creates flexibility, tendons and ligaments have very little and by design do not stretch well. Bone itself is living tissue covered by a smooth layer of connective tissue with a dense layer of compact bone underneath. The deepest layer is spongy bone made of a matrix, making bones strong and light. Weight-bearing exercise improves bone density, which protects bones from breaking under impact, stress, and the unpredictable stuff that happens out in the wild.

Connective tissue is strong and forms the ligaments and tendons as well as the fascia. Fascia is woven connective tissue that wraps around all muscles, creating a weave that can stick together similar to something getting caught in a web. It is not just a system of separate coverings. It is actually one continuous structure that exists from head to toe without interruption. It covers and interpenetrates every muscle, bone, nerve, artery, and vein, as well as all of our internal organs including the heart, lungs, brain, and spinal cord.

Muscular Engagement

We know that muscles contract and relax, but it is important to note the different types of muscular engagement as we move forward through anatomy, alignment, and practice. Contraction of a muscle that shortens the distance between the two joints, such as engaging the biceps, which bends your elbow, is called **concentric contraction**. **Eccentric contraction** happens when the muscle engaged lengthens, the way the biceps muscle contracts but lengthens to straighten the elbow. When muscle length remains the same during engagement, it is known as **isometric contraction**. All types of muscle contraction occur throughout *asana* practice to move in and out of postures. Isometric contraction happens when we hold postures for a prolonged time, such as five breaths or more. As you read through the

" YOGA PHILOSOPHY VIEWS THE WHOLE BODY AS A DYNAMIC AND COMPLEX SYSTEM—EVERYTHING AFFECTING EVERYTHING ELSE—AND AIMS TO CREATE INTEGRATION."

SKELETAL SYSTEM

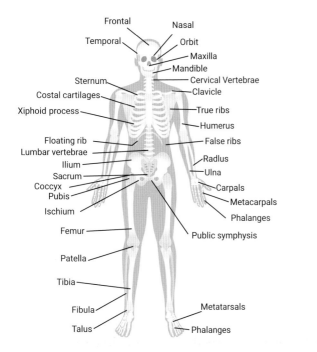

Frontal
Nasal
Temporal
Orbit
Maxilla
Mandible
Sternum
Cervical Vertebrae
Costal cartilages
Clavicle
Xiphoid process
True ribs
Humerus
Floating rib
False ribs
Lumbar vertebrae
Ilium
Radlus
Sacrum
Ulna
Coccyx
Carpals
Pubis
Metacarpals
Ischium
Phalanges
Femur
Public symphysis
Patella
Tibia
Fibula
Metatarsals
Talus
Phalanges

MUSCULAR SYSTEM

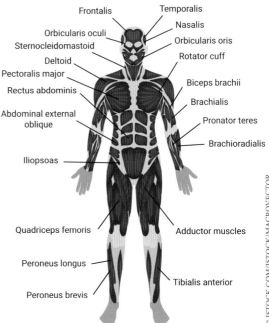

Frontalis
Temporalis
Nasalis
Orbicularis oculi
Orbicularis oris
Sternocleidomastoid
Rotator cuff
Deltoid
Pectoralis major
Biceps brachii
Rectus abdominis
Brachialis
Abdominal external
oblique
Pronator teres
Brachioradialis
Iliopsoas
Quadriceps femoris
Adductor muscles
Peroneus longus
Tibialis anterior
Peroneus brevis

anatomy, alignment, and *asana* chapters, the instructions are mainly focused on external cues to help create muscle engagement, such as pulling back on your heels when in bridge pose to isometrically contract the hamstrings. As you practice, you can use these refinements of engagement to deepen your experience of the postures.

Spine

The spine is the center of the body and yoga practices. The spine is made up of thirty-three vertebrae—seven cervical, twelve thoracic, and five lumbar—along with the sacrum (five fused sacral vertebrae) and the coccyx (four frequently fused coccygeal vertebrae). These interconnected bones support the brain and house the spinal cord, the central information system of the body. All the sensory input from every nerve in the body travels through the spine to communicate with the brain. Yoga philosophy views the spine as the superhighway of the subtle channels connecting us to ourselves and the world around us.

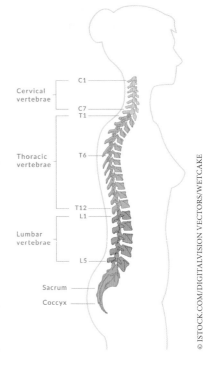

Cervical
vertebrae
C1
C7
T1
Thoracic
vertebrae
T6
T12
L1
Lumbar
vertebrae
L5
Sacrum
Coccyx

Keeping the spine healthy allows for free flow of energy and information. Spinal health is one of the most powerful aspects of yoga, encouraging and sustaining balance, mobility, and support.

There are four main curves of the spine. The cervical spine moves in a lordotic (anterior) curve toward the front of the body. The thoracic spine moves in a kyphotic (posterior) curve toward the back body. The lumbar is lordotic and the sacrum is kyphotic. Neutral curves in the spine create the most stable and mobile structure, while extreme curvature of the thoracic, known as kyphosis, creates a hunch in the upper back with considerable strain on the neck (think tech neck). Lordosis is an exaggerated curvature of the lumbar that creates a swayback, putting excess pressure on the low back.

Feet/Ankles

Human feet are quite complex and amazing. As we evolved from four to two feet, the shape and size of the foot bones had to change. There are twenty-six bones and thirty-three joints in each foot. The calcaneus (heel bone) and the talus (which sits just above the heel) form the base of the foot and carry most of the weight. The talus connects the tibia and fibula (shin bones) to form the ankle joint. Five small interlocking tarsal bones connect the calcaneus to the toes, allowing for greater mobility of the feet, which improves balance and strength up the body. Three main ligaments form the arches: the medial, lateral, and transverse. Arches act as shock absorbers and are important to the alignment, function, and support of the rest of the body.

The ankle is a hinge joint that can be flexed to draw the toes toward the shin (dorsiflexion), or pointed to extend the front of the ankle (plantarflexion). Eversion (sole of the foot moves away from the centerline of the body) and inversion (sole of the food moves toward the centerline) are movements within the foot itself. **Tibialis anterior** is a larger muscle that runs down the front of the shin bone and creates dorsiflexion of the foot. The **peroneal** muscles run along the outside of the shin and help stabilize the outer ankle. On the back of the lower leg are the calf muscles: **gastrocnemius** and **soleus**. Both of these muscles point the ankle and assist in walking, jumping, and stabilizing the knee.

Knees/Thighs

The knee is a hinge joint that flexes (bends the knee) and extends (straightens the knee). It is composed of the top of the tibia and fibula, the patella, and the lower femur bone and ligaments that surround the knee joint. Two fibrocartilage discs sit atop the the tibia, creating cushion for the knee. The tibial collateral ligament, patellar ligament, medial collateral ligament, and lateral collateral ligament support the exterior of the knee joint, while the anterior cruciate and posterior cruciate ligaments stabilize the knee from within. The patella is contained within the patellar ligament, which is formed by the ends of the quadriceps muscles and attaches to the front and top of the tibia bone. The knee can rotate slightly when bent, but twisting a straight knee can cause acute knee injuries. Uneven surfaces on backcountry trails and slopes sometimes demand rotation of the knee with no warning. Practicing body awareness and alignment through yoga helps prepare the body for rigorous adventure. Yoga can shorten the body's response time, giving you a chance to react to surprise obstacles in your path and by engaging supporting muscles to maintain balance.

The femur, or thigh bone, is the largest bone in the body and connects two of our most consequential joints—the hips and the knee. Numerous muscle groups, tendons, and ligaments cross over these joints and connect to the femur. The **quadriceps** is the large group of muscles on the front of the thigh bone with converging sections that connect the front of the hip to the knee. The four muscles constituting the quadriceps are the rectus femoris, vastus intermedius, vastus lateralis, and vastus medialis. **Rectus femoris** is the only muscle that crosses the hip and the knee joint, and acts to flex the hip and extend the knee. **Vastus intermedius** is the smaller muscle at the top of the thigh bone, while **vastus lateralis** and **vastus medialis** are on either side of the front of the thigh bone. When the quadriceps muscles engage they extend the knee, straightening the leg. They are engaged when we walk, run, hike, ski, bike, and climb. Stretching these muscles through yoga poses, including low lunge, lizard lunge, and hero pose, balances that strength with flexibility, which helps in recovery and performance. The **sartorius** muscle is the longest in the body and crosses the hip and knee joints. It flexes, laterally rotates, and abducts the hip and flexes the knee. It is often restricted in cyclists, hikers, paddlers, and snowboarders, while skiers and climbers often have more flexibility in this muscle due to increased abduction (moving the legs away from the midline). Practicing yoga postures such as warrior two, *skandasana*, frog pose, and cobbler's pose improves the flexibility of the sartorius.

The **hamstrings** are located behind the thigh bone and contract to flex the knee. They attach at the sit bones (ischial tuberosities) and insert below and on the sides of the knee. The three muscles from the midline outward are the **semimembranosus**, the **biceps femoris**, and the **semitendinosus**. On the inside (medial) of the thigh bone are the **adductors**, which bring the leg inward toward the midline of the body. The **pectineus**, **adductor brevis**, and **adductor longus** attach to the pubic bone of the pelvis and insert along the upper inner thigh. **Gracilis** is long and thin, running from the back of the pubic bone to just below the knee, and the **adductor magnus** is the strongest adductor, running from the sit bone to the back of the thigh bone.

Hips

Numerous muscles attach to the hips and provide both range of motion and stability of this ball-and-socket joint. Formed by the top of the femur (thigh bone) and the hollow space of the pelvis called the acetabulum, the joint is secured by ligaments, tendons, and muscle. There are six lateral rotators of the thigh bone: **piriformis**, **obturator internus**, **obturator externus**, **gemellus superior**, **gemellus inferior**, and **quadratus femoris**. **Psoas major** is the main trunk and hip flexor and the culprit of much low back and knee pain. It resides deep within the core and joins with the **iliacus**. The three **gluteal** muscles are the primary stabilizers and movers for extension and lateral rotation of the hip. **Gluteus medius**, **gluteus maximus**, and **gluteus minimus** extend the hip and assist in abduction and medial rotation of the thigh and lateral flexion of the pelvis.

Tensor fascia latae begins at the front and top of the pelvis and runs along the outside, inserting into the iliotibial tract, or IT band. Another important hip and trunk flexor is the **iliopsoas** (iliacus plus psoas major). It runs deep under the abdominal muscles from the lower ribs, along the sides of the lumbar spine, and through the pelvis and attaches at the upper inner thigh bone. It plays a vital role in pelvic movement and the curvature of the lower spine. On either side of the sacrum, the large triangular-shaped bone that functions as the keystone of the pelvis, are the sacroiliac joints. There is very little movement here, yet dysfunction and imbalances are common causes for low back pain.

Torso/Core

As the central axis of the body housing the spine, the torso has a fairly large range of motion. Let's look at the muscles along the back chain of the body. Deepest along the spine originate the **erector spinae**, which stabilize from the skull down to the pelvis. The **trapezius**, **rhomboids**, **serratus anterior**, and **latissimus dorsi** help stabilize the shoulders and are superficial (closer to the skin) than the erectors. Closer to the pelvis lies the **quadratus lumborum**, running from the lower ribs along the lumbar spine and attaching to the top of the hip at the pelvic crest. Supporting small muscles called the **multifidi** run along the lower spine, attaching to the top of the sacrum and iliac crest, and assist in supporting the lumbar curve.

On the front of the torso we find **pectoralis major** and **minor** on the chest, which adduct the upper arm bone. The **abdominals** including the **external oblique**, **internal oblique**, **transverse abdominis**, and **rectus abdominis** stretch from the lower sternum and ribs and run along the front of the torso. These stabilize and protect the vital organs, ribs, and the spine. Underneath the abdominals are the **psoas major** and **iliacus** mentioned above, which flex the trunk and the hip.

Shoulders/Arms

The shoulder is made up of the articulation of the upper arm bone, the scapula (shoulder blade), the clavicle (collarbone), and the sternum (breastbone). The main joint is the glenohumeral joint between the head of the humerus (upper arm bone) and the hollow of the glenoid fossa of the scapula. A ball-and-socket joint similar to the hip joint, the glenohumeral joint is more shallow and with fewer attachments. Greater range of motion means less stability, meaning the shoulder is vulnerable to dislocation. The two other joints of the shoulder are the acromioclavicular joint, between the outer end of the clavicle and the acromion process of the scapula (top outer point), and the sternoclavicular joint attaching the collarbone to the breastbone. In essence, the shoulders are very free, only attaching to the central skeleton at the breastbone.

Movements of the shoulder at the scapula include elevation, depression, protraction (moving away from the spine), retraction (moving toward the spine), upward rotation (lower scapula toward the midline), and downward rotation (lower scapula away from the midline). These movements assist with movements of the upper arm bone (humerus) to flex, extend, and abduct the arm. Movements of the upper arm include adduction, abduction, internal and external rotation, flexion, and extension.

Let's look at the four **rotator cuff** muscles first. The **subscapularis** attaches on the medial border of the scapula, covering it and connecting to the back of the top of the humerus. It creates medial rotation and adduction of the arm. **Infraspinatus** lies under the subscapularis, attaching at the medial border of the scapula and at the back of the upper humerus, rotating laterally. Sitting on the upper portion of the scapula is the **supraspinatus**. It attaches at the top of the humerus and abducts the arm (lifting away from the midline). Lastly, **teres minor** attaches at the outer, lower edge of the scapula, inserting at the top of the humerus, which assists in lateral rotation. These four muscles create stability around the scapula and upper arm bone.

Continuing with the back of the shoulder is the **serratus anterior**. It is a broad muscle that covers the outer rib cage and inserts on the front side of the scapula, helping stabilize the shoulder blades. It creates protraction and rotation of the scapula and is used in pushing motions. The **rhomboids** (major and minor) attach to the inner border of the scapula, connecting to the last cervical vertebra and the first five thoracic vertebrae. They assist in downward rotation and adduction. Another stabilizing muscle is the **levator scapulae**, which attaches at the upper medial edge of the scapula, connecting to the first four cervical vertebrae. It elevates and rotates downward. The large diamond-shaped muscle that overlays these deeper muscles is the **trapezius**. It begins at the occiput (base of skull) and continues down to the last thoracic vertebra. It inserts on the spine of the scapula, creating retraction (toward the spine). The upper fibers create elevation and upward rotation of the scapula, the lower fibers create depression, and both upper and lower fibers create upward rotation. **Triceps brachii** lies on the back of the upper arm bone and extends as well as assists with adduction.

Moving to the side of the shoulder, we find the **deltoid** at the top of the upper arm bone. It is the round shape of the outer shoulder and creates a cap between the scapula, collarbone, and humerus. It acts to abduct the arm, but the frontal deltoid fibers also create flexion and medial rotation. The back of the deltoid fibers assist in extension and internal rotation. In the front plane of the body is the **biceps brachii**, which originates at the outer edge of the scapula, the coracoid process, and the head of the humerus. Attaching at the medial forearm creates flexion and supination (turning the palm upward) of the forearm as well as abduction and adduction. One last primary shoulder muscle connects to the skull and is part of the neck. The **sternocleidomastoid** mainly moves the head, but will elevate the clavicle if the head is stationary. It also assists in inhalation.

Lower Arms/Hands

From yoga to climbing and paddling, nearly every activity requires our hands. To begin to understand the anatomy of the hands and wrists, let's start farther up with the radius and ulna bones. These two bones of the forearm create the elbow joint along with the humerus (upper arm bone). The elbow is a hinge joint moving between flexion (hand toward bicep) and extension (straight arm). The elbow often hyperextends in hypermobile bodies, similar to the knee joint. Similarly, keeping the joint soft helps keep it aligned when straight and encourages surrounding muscles to engage. **Biceps brachii** and **brachioradialis** flex the elbow, while the triceps extend it.

The forearm has two movements—supination turns the palm upward, while pronation turns the palm downward (thumb closer to the body). During these movements the radius crosses and uncrosses the ulna. Climbing and other daily activities place a great deal of strain on these muscles. **Pronator teres** pronates the forearm, while **brachioradialis** assists in supination.

At the wrist joint, the radius articulates with the carpal bones, small bones similar to those in the foot. Beyond the carpal bones are the metacarpals, which make up the palm of the hand, and the phalanges, which are the finger bones. One area to note is the carpal joint and the carpal tunnel. This area can become tight due to underuse or overuse of the hand. While practicing *asana* helps support the wrist joint, variations that are less weight bearing on the hands may be helpful at first (especially for climbers).

RESPIRATORY ANATOMY

The respiratory system includes the nasal cavities, air passageway tubes (larynx and trachea), and lungs. Humans take fifteen to twenty breaths per minute on average, oxygenating cells and ridding the body of carbon dioxide. Respiration is part of the autonomic nervous system, and breathing happens automatically. The diaphragm is a dome-shaped muscle that attaches to the back of the spine and circles around the bottom of the ribs to the xiphoid process at the base of the sternum. It separates the upper organs from the abdominal organs and assists breathing. When we inhale, the diaphragm drops, creating negative pressure and drawing air into the lungs. When we exhale, the diaphragm relaxes and the rib cage compresses, releasing air. Belly breathing and breathing with *bandhas* (locks of pressure) are explained in the Yoga of Breathing chapter.

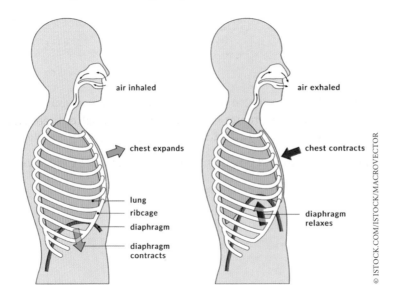

For our purposes it is important to understand that the musculature of the torso and upper body influence breathing patterns, as does postural alignment. If you tend to be a shallow breather, your shoulders and spine can round forward, further restricting the breath. If your core and upper body are well developed from activities such as climbing and paddling, tension in the **pectoralis** muscles and **abdominal** muscles can restrict your breathing. Small muscles that run between the ribs called **intercostals** may also be restricted, reducing the rib cage and lungs' ability to expand. Lastly, the alignment of the neck and balance of muscle tension can restrict the entry of breath. Notice how your breath changes when you move your head forward and upward versus sliding the top of the throat back and lowering the chin slightly.

THE TAKEAWAY

While this may feel like a lot of biological and technical information, it is so helpful in understanding what is going on with your body. Understanding anatomy may or may not come easy for you, but since you have a human body, having a basic understanding of the musculoskeletal system is empowering. It will also help you understand patterns and unlock the potential in the practices of yoga. The main points to take away are:

- The whole body functions together, and the musculoskeletal system affects every other system.

- The musculoskeletal system is connected by a vast network of connective tissue, bone, and muscle. Fascia is a living system covering every muscle in the body.

- Muscles are attached to tendons, which attach to bones. Therefore, when muscles are tight or habitually contracted, they pull on other muscles, tendons, and bones.

- Yoga helps create more balance between the entire musculoskeletal system as well as greater body awareness and better breathing, and trains the nervous system to relax the body more efficiently.

- Muscle tension and postural alignment affect our ability to breath properly.

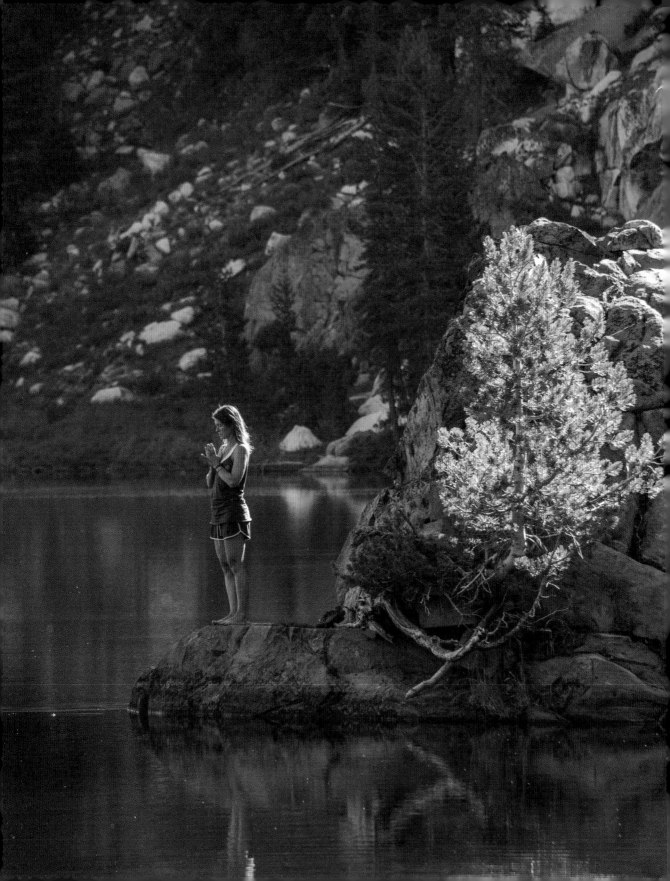

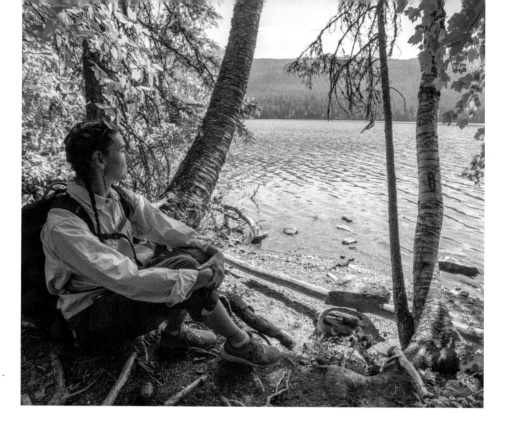

CHAPTER 3

ALIGNMENT PRINCIPLES

Our dream is to have all of us moving sure-footedly through our forests—be they of wood, of steel and concrete, or of humanity.
—R. LOUIS SCHULTZ, PHD, AND ROSEMARY FEITIS,
DOCTOR OF OSTEOPATHY

OVER THE LAST TWENTY YEARS OF PRACTICING AND STUDYING yoga, massage, and Ayurveda, I have seen definitions of alignment evolve. With the increase in functional movement research, there has been a shift in the yoga community to look more deeply at what alignment means and what the goal of practicing *asana* is. Moving away from rigid adherence to traditional alignment in a posture, there is a growing interest in personalizing postures to meet an individual's needs. A beautifully expressed pose may be more harmful than beneficial if it involves overextension or patterns prone to overuse injuries. Traditionally impeccable practices may not be sustainable for some bodies if done repeatedly over time and may not be suitable for someone with injuries or after surgery. For example, it may be more beneficial to keep the back knee down in a lunge pose to lengthen the hip flexors, as opposed to straightening the back leg and hyperextending the low back. In revolved triangle it might be better to allow some hip rotation instead of keeping the hips square, to take pressure off the sacroiliac joint and deepen release in the outer hip muscles. Most important is to start where you are and work with the body you have. Everyone can practice yoga, but postures will look different for different people.

Traditionally, alignment cues have been very universal, seeking to create an external shape of alignment rather than a personalized internal alignment. There are wide variations in the shapes of the pelvis, curvatures of the spine, and shapes of joints such as the shoulder or hip. Often alignment cues have focused on the extremities first and core last. Cues for standing poses often begin by aligning the feet symmetrically with outer edges parallel, and aligning the hands with middle fingers parallel is the baseline for downward facing dog pose. Students are often instructed to align the rest of the body from this fixed position without accounting for individual physical needs and history. Practicing this external and so-called universal alignment over and over again, however, may strain many students' knees, hips, spine, and upper body. Asymmetry is more common than symmetry, in my experience, and attempting to force symmetry can lead to injury and interfere with daily activities and adventures. Aligning from the core of the body—pelvis up to the head—creates more stability and greater mobility. This approach often leads to more symmetry in the periphery (hands and feet) and fewer injuries. We all have different physical histories, and there is huge variation in our bone and joint structures. Trying to fit into an external blueprint is not the goal of yoga. Instead of forcing your body into poses, allow the poses to develop from internal alignment of the core and practice with patience, kindness, and honesty.

Keep in mind this is an emerging way of practicing and teaching yoga. Most likely you have been or will be taught these external principles of aligning hands and feet in certain ways. I encourage you to carefully explore your personal needs and deeply respect the feedback your body and nervous system give you. If you feel pain in any joint, back off. Try a different alignment of the feet or hands and go back to the internal alignment of your torso. Keep this in mind as you look at classes and teachers. Do some research into their background and approach, interview them, and discuss your individual needs before you take a class. It is good and healthy to practice discernment. You know your body best. An experienced yoga teacher will be open to helping you find what works for you.

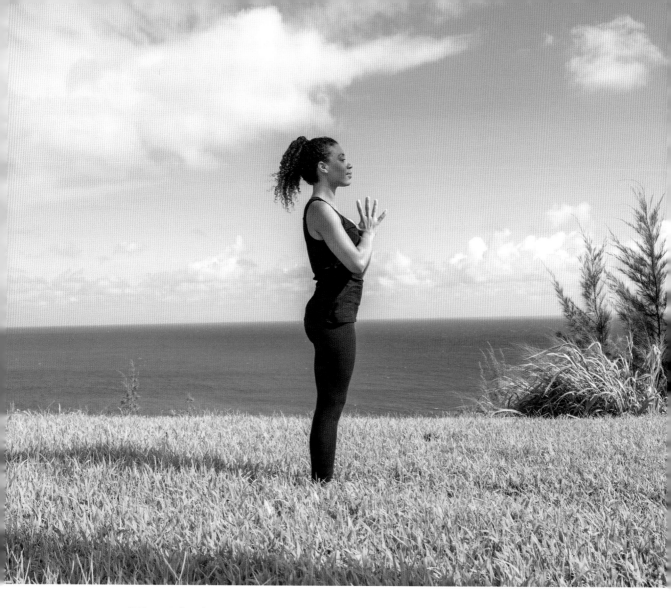

When I first began practicing yoga in 1999, my personal goal was to reduce pain and improve my posture. I have spent most of my yoga career practicing and studying alignment-based yoga, using props to support my spinal alignment, which has improved immensely. The foundational postures, which once felt like torture, are deeply releasing and comfortable now. As I began to work on deeper postures and variations over the years, I realized I still held compensation patterns that needed to be addressed. In 2008, a low back injury sent me to find an experienced physical therapist, and I began to slowly retrain my movement patterns and alignment. Practicing yoga is now a journey of experimentation, research, and deeper listening to my body with more *ahimsa* and respect.

" INSTEAD OF FORCING YOUR BODY INTO POSES, ALLOW THE POSES TO DEVELOP FROM INTERNAL ALIGNMENT OF THE CORE AND PRACTICE WITH PATIENCE, KINDNESS, AND HONESTY."

Like many athletes, I was used to pushing my body toward physical goals and enduring various pains. In my *asana* practice this looked like overstretching ligaments and hyperextending my spine in order to "go deeper." Learning how to walk again post-injury was a humbling experience that heightened my awareness of alignment and balance. Walking in nature connects me to my truth and to something far greater and magnificent. Humbly, I began to reassess my intentions around my yoga practice and how it fit into the greater picture of my life. Nagging knee and back pain had kept me from enjoying many outdoor activities that bring me so much happiness. I wanted my yoga practice to support the whole of my life, not take it over at the expense of my love of the outdoors. My approach to my practice changed, and the goals were different. I stripped my practices down to those I knew I needed for addressing structural imbalances, breathing practices, and meditation. Slowly a deeper and more stable internal alignment developed. Working consistently within my safe range of motion has expanded my movement potential and sustainability. Nowadays my practice is focused on equal parts strength, stability, and mobility. The alignment principles in this book are geared toward functional movement and sustainability to enjoy a healthy life outdoors. I encourage you to explore alignment and variations in postures to find what feels best in your body and for your personal needs. Big, beautiful poses are great, but what's the point if they compromise your structural integrity and negatively affect your outdoor passions?

ACTIVE FEET

Since the feet are our primary foundation in movement of any kind, we want to begin aligning from the ground up. Let's first look at how our feet are aligned habitually. With bare feet, walk in place for about 20 seconds without trying to "do" anything about alignment. When you stop moving, stand with your eyes closed for another 10 seconds or more. Notice how your weight is balanced on each foot—heels or front of the foot? Inside or outside of the foot? How does the weight distribution differ from left to right foot? Then open your eyes and look down without moving your feet. Notice if one foot is in front of the other, or if one or both are turned outward or inward. Just notice the patterns.

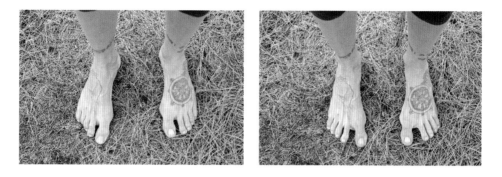

Now step your feet apart about one foot length. Spread your toes, keeping your big toes grounded. This will activate the arches of your feet, widen your base, and engage the muscles. Balance the weight between your feet left to right and front to back. Press through the mound of the big toe, the mound of the little toe, and the center of your heel. Press down evenly through your feet, activating them and your lower leg muscles. Take a few breaths here and feel the engagement. In yoga this is called *pada bandha* (foot lock), which creates a firm rooting to the earth, activates the arches, and creates a lifting of muscles upward through the body. Creating this foot engagement in all standing postures and as much as possible in other activities helps set a strong and grounded foundation for the rest of the body.

KNEES

Knee alignment is directly influenced by the alignment of the ankle below and pelvis above. Chronic locking of the knees can stress the ligaments of the joint and lead to a greater risk of ligament damage and other injuries like a Baker's cyst (swelling and pain behind the knee). This pattern also encourages the heads of the femur bones to push forward, creating imbalance in the low back and core. When the thigh bones move forward habitually, the head of the bone moves away from the deep socket, placing stress on the stabilizing ligaments and increasing risk of injury.

To activate and align the knees, start by grounding your feet—balancing your weight evenly and softening your knees. Slowly contract your thigh muscles, lifting your kneecaps and pulling the top of the thigh bones up and back slightly. Repeat this exercise a few times and notice when you've gone too far, hyperextending the knees, losing the tone of the thighs, and pushing the top of the thigh bones forward. If you have been locking your knees most of your life, you will feel as though your legs aren't straight when your knees are properly aligned. It will take practice and patience to retrain the thigh muscles and build kinesthetic awareness.

Lastly, the knees should be facing forward when standing. The knee is a hinge joint and is safest (when weight bearing) aligning with the toes instead of turning outward or inward. When the legs are fully engaged and the knees are not locked,

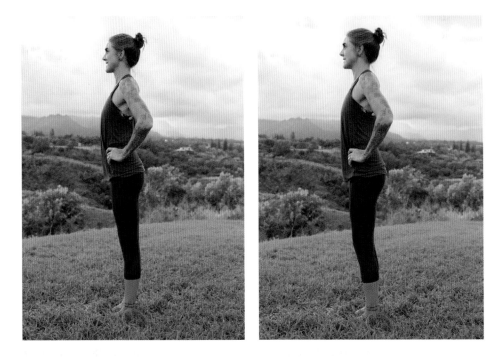

the direction the knees face may be affected by the alignment of the feet. For some people, aligning the feet so the big toes touch and there is space between the heels will help turn the knees straight ahead. For others, this action may turn the knees inward, weakening the inner ligaments. Try aligning your feet so the inner edges are parallel and notice if your knees now face forward. You may even have one foot that needs to turn out a little more than the other for both knees to face forward. Practice these different cues to see what works best for your body.

NEUTRAL PELVIS

Let's review some key bony landmarks for reference before we get into the alignment of the pelvis. On either side of the front of your hips are two bony points, the anterior superior iliac spine (ASIS). From the back of your pelvis on either side of your sacrum (the large triangular bone at base of spine) are two bony points called the posterior superior iliac spine (PSIS). These are the landmarks we use when finding a neutral pelvic alignment. If we draw a line between the ASIS and PSIS from a side view, it shows the angle of the pelvis. For most men it will be around 0 degrees when neutral, while for most women it averages around 15 degrees. Bear in mind there are wide variations among male and female pelvis shapes and angles. Genetics and tensional patterns can create larger or smaller angles between the ASIS and the PSIS. Another cue for finding a neutral pelvis is lining up the ASIS with the pubic bone on the vertical plane.

To find your neutral pelvis, go back to setting the feet and knees first, drawing the inner thighs and tops of the thigh bones back just slightly as you engage the legs and lower belly. The back of the legs, gluteal muscles, and abdominal muscles will all be engaged slightly when you find neutral without the low back tightening or front ribs popping forward. Use a mirror as reference and turn to the side. Align the center of your ear, middle of the upper arm bone, midpoint of the hip bone, and the midline of the heel vertically. Use this as reference when standing, exercising, practicing yoga, and sitting.

In seated postures you use the sit bones (ischial tuberosities) as your foundation instead of the feet. Continue to keep the feet and legs engaged to help align the pelvis. You can rock forward and backward on your sit bones, noticing how it affects the spinal alignment as you move. Then find a neutral position in the pelvis by weighting the sit bones evenly from front to back and side to side. If your low back tends to round, sitting on a blanket, towel, or rolled-up jacket (great when practicing outdoors) works well to lift the hips and encourage a neutral tilt to the pelvis.

The pelvis moves dynamically in the course of sports and yoga practice. When running, hiking, climbing, cycling, etc., the pelvis tends to tip forward when the legs or back are extended. Likewise while climbing or seated in a canoe, kayak, or on a bike, the pelvis tends to tuck under when the legs or spine are flexed. As you move through a range of motions, the actions required for leveling the pelvis change. While standing the actions are subtle. When you move into standing forward fold, you lengthen the sit bones upward and draw the belly inward to keep the spine in an even curve. In postures that extend the legs or back, such as lunges, warrior one, warrior two, and all backbending poses, the actions need to be stronger by rooting the sit bones downward and lifting the lower belly upward to create a more neutral pelvic tilt. A common and helpful image is to see your pelvis as a bowl holding water. We want to keep the water in the bowl with all of our movements.

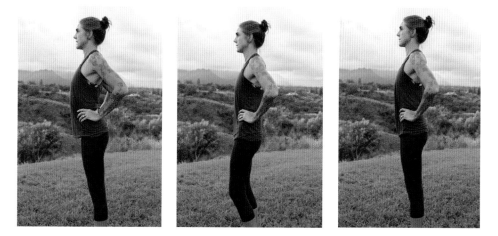

RIBS IN

A common pattern for many people is to lift the floating ribs upward when trying to stand up straight, engaging the shoulders or backbending. If you are not sure if this is you, try this: Stand perpendicular to a mirror. Glance at your spinal curvature, rib cage, and height while standing naturally, then look forward. Stand up straight and apply what you know as good posture, then take another look in the mirror. Have you actually gotten any taller? Is your lordotic curve more pronounced? Can you see your bottom ribs lifting up and away from the top of your abdomen? If so, start to expand your understanding of good posture to include the relationship of your upper body to your mid-body.

Puffing the ribs up and away from the core weakens the upper abdominal muscles, tightens the low back muscles, and reduces the breath capacity. When you set the foundation of the feet, legs, hips, and core, it becomes much easier to find a neutral position for the rib cage. Keeping this foundation, try to breathe into the back of your rib cage, allowing it to expand backward. This helps loosen the muscles between the ribs, which are often restricted, and helps align the rib cage, drawing the lower front ribs inward. Knit your front ribs together on the exhalation, engaging your upper abdominal muscles slightly. When either bending backward in spinal extension or folding forward in hip flexion, on a bike or in a canoe, we want to maintain this action as much as possible to support the breath, the core, and the low back. As with pelvic alignment, maintaining neutral rib positioning requires more strength as range of motion increases.

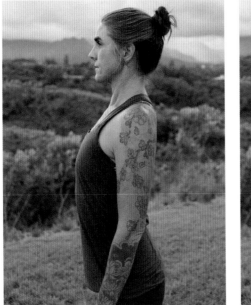 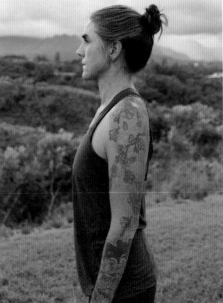

SHOULDERS

The shoulder girdle (scapula, collarbones, and sternum) rests on the rib cage and only attaches to the central skeleton at the sternum. Unlike the pelvis, which is anchored to the spine at the sacrum, the shoulder girdle has much greater range of motion but also less stability. Since it rests on the rib cage, the breath has a great impact on shoulder alignment. If your breath is normally shallow or you breathe primarily from your belly, the upper rib cage and shoulders will be more restricted in movement and have less support. If you breathe into the front of the body normally, then the upper spine (thoracic) and scapula may be restricted. Working on expanding your breathing into the back, sides, and top of the rib cage will help improve shoulder alignment and stability throughout your activities and daily life.

Most arm and shoulder movements happen in front of the body, which means the muscles of the chest (pectoral) and shoulders (anterior deltoid and serratus anterior) tend to be stronger than those in the back of the shoulders (rhomboids, latissimus dorsi). This moves the head of the arm bone (humerus) forward and out of the stability of the glenohumeral joint (shoulder). Depending on your activities this can increase the risk of a shoulder dislocation or rotator cuff injury.

Optimal alignment for the shoulders is to draw the tops of the shoulders down away from the ears and draw the scapula toward the spine slightly. Full breathing naturally supports this lifting of the sternum. Try to maintain a slight engagement of the shoulders drawing back toward the spine and downward when reaching the arms

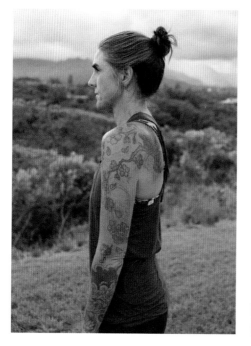 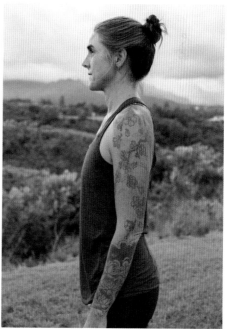

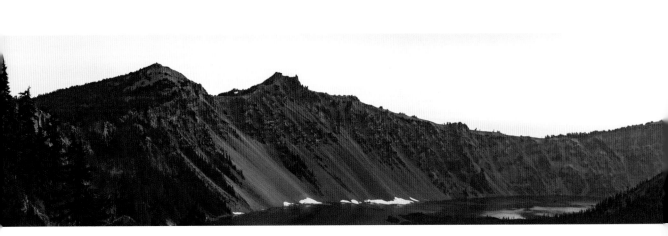

forward. While pushing through the hands, keep the tops of the shoulders drawing downward and widen the scapula. When reaching up and pulling downward in climbing or paddling, try to maintain the pull of the shoulder blades downward and engage the latissimus dorsi muscles while lifting the top of the sternum. All of these actions help stabilize the shoulder girdle while active in sports and in yoga.

ACTIVE HANDS

Whether you are a climber, cyclist, paddler, or skier, most outdoor athletes have strong hands and grip. All that gripping can lead to tight hands and wrists and tension in the forearms. Working on wrist mobility and stability is key for the health not just of the hands but also the elbows and shoulders. Stretching the fingers wide balances the muscles of the wrist and forearm and helps engage the biceps and triceps.

Try relaxing your hands and feel the muscle tension in your arms and shoulders. Now spread your fingers wide apart and press into the fingertips, feeling the muscular engagement of the entire arm into the shoulder. Practice this action whenever your hands are on the mat and when your arms are outstretched in postures like warrior one and two. This action will balance the strength of the entire arm and help take pressure off the wrists and elbows while practicing yoga.

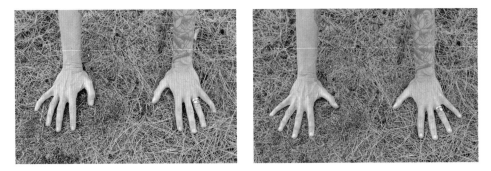

NECK

The neck consists of the seven cervical vertebrae and has a greater range of motion than the rest of the spine. This makes it more flexible and more vulnerable. Commonly people have too much curve in the cervical spine from poor postural habits and too much sitting. This puts pressure on the discs and increases neck tension that translates into the muscles of the head. To remedy the head forward and chin up position, move the top of the throat back and lengthen up through the back of the head. Lift upward through the crown of the head to create space between the vertebrae and around the base of the skull. Lastly, relax the jaw muscles, letting the bottom row of teeth release from the top and allowing the neck muscles to lengthen.

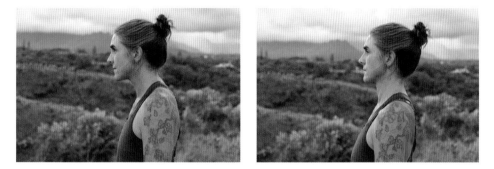

THE TAKEAWAY

Athletes tend to be pretty hard on their bodies through training, competing, and playing. Even small habitual misalignments of the joints and spine increase the risk of injury and chronic pain. Your yoga practice is a time to slow down, to pay attention to your body moving in space, and to align your body and breath in ways that support healing and resiliency.

- Use these alignment principles while practicing yoga and throughout the rest of your activities.

- These alignment cues are often subtle shifts, increasing body awareness and breathing patterns.

- More weight bearing and greater challenge require a stronger action to maintain optimal alignment.

- Outdoor sports and yoga are dynamic expressions of life, harmony, and disharmony. Alignment awareness helps us tune into the interconnectedness of nature.

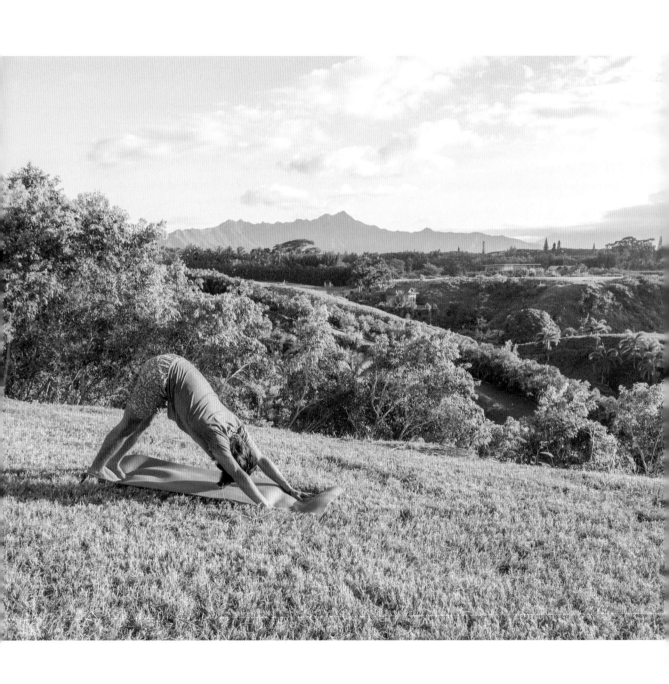

YOGI INSIGHT

NOELL CLARK

E-RYT 500 yoga coach for San Francisco 49ers, instructor and
yoga teacher trainer for Breathe Together Yoga; San Jose, CA.

What changes are you seeing in the world of alignment as you teach?
I'm seeing a bigger focus on looking at the whole person. There are so many different bodies and stories that show up to class, and they all have different patterns from life. I see people holding the old pattern of constantly retracting and depressing their shoulders in standing poses, for one. With this alignment, if you have more of an anterior tilt to your pelvis, especially for women, then the pelvis will always have a swayback and the ribs will always pop forward. Another is the shift to focusing on building strength in the posterior chain of the body. It clears up so many issues.

How has this shift changed your focus in teaching?
Instead of poses I teach body movement mechanics. I have done more training in functional range conditioning (FRC) and the Eldoa Method. My classes are focused on teaching small somatic exercises and then postures.

What are the biggest things you see athletes needing from yoga?
Yoga helps them rehabilitate an injury by mobilizing an area and slowly increasing the load (weight or resistance). Secondly, It gives them tools to tap into the parasympathetic system, since they are so often chronically in the sympathetic response of fight or flight. Integrating better breathing into their daily life has been a game changer. Incorporating internal rotation of the legs helps them offset the outer rotation dominance of their sports and helps with spinal decompression. All of this helps them find ease during challenges and improves their performance.

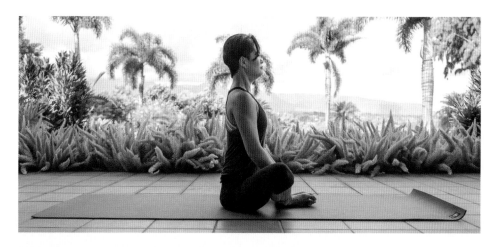

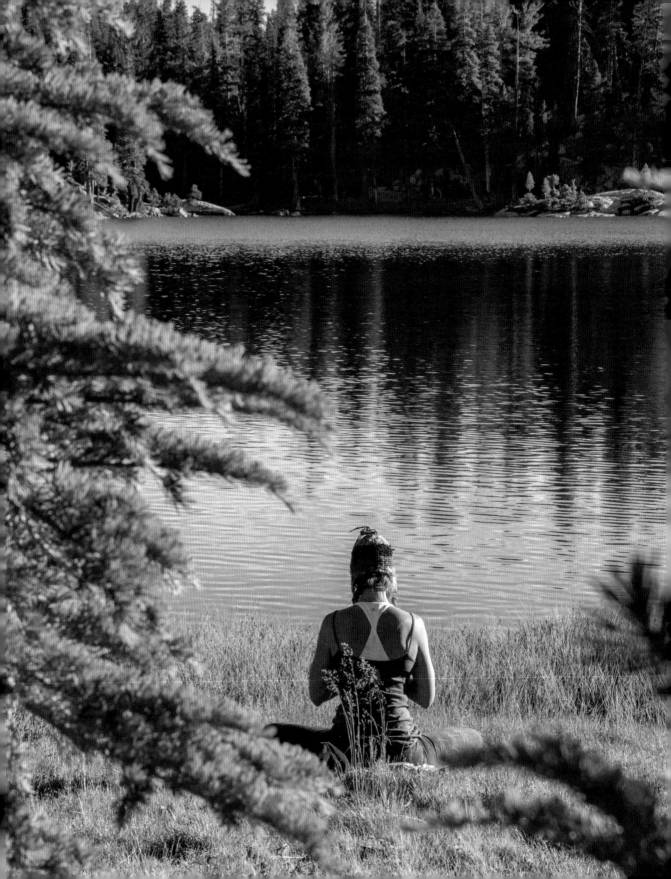

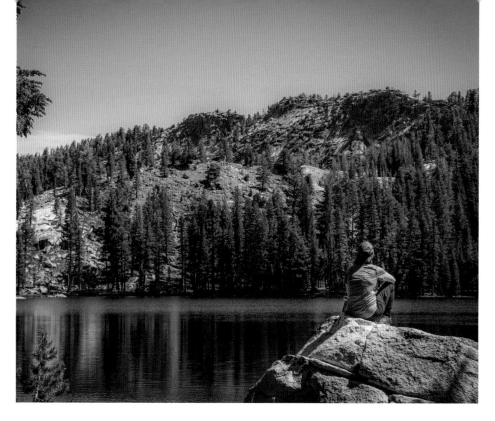

CHAPTER 4

YOGA OF BREATHING

When the breath wanders the mind also is unsteady. But when the breath is calmed the mind too will be still, and the yogi achieves a long life. Therefore, one should learn to control the breath.

—SVATMARAMA, HATHA YOGA PRADIPIKA

ANCIENT YOGIS AND MODERN SCIENCE SHOW US that when we consciously attend to our breathing patterns we can directly affect the nervous system and therefore the entire body and mind. Learning to breathe consciously is one of the most profound benefits of practicing yoga. The average person takes more than 20,000 breaths per day, providing lots of opportunity to practice and make the most of our breath. Breath is life, and by improving our breathing we unlock what yogis call *prana*, life force energy. *Asana* practice is essentially a breathing practice as we move our bodies through space into different shapes and relationships to gravity. We have discussed how *asana* practice helps improve muscular and postural balance and improves our breath capacity. By engaging with all eight limbs on a daily basis, we can bring the practice into all areas of our lives. And what is more constant in life than breathing?

To begin, start to become aware of your natural breathing pattern. Lie on your back with your knees bent, feet flat on the floor about hip distance apart. Place your hands on your belly. Relax everything else and let the ground support you. A folded blanket or thin pillow under the back of your head can offset any neck strain you may feel. Just breathe. Begin to notice where you feel the inhalation the most—perhaps in your belly, your chest, or your back. Just notice. Then begin to notice the quality of your inhalation—its length, restrictions, sound, and depth. Next, focus on your exhalation, noting where you feel it begin, where you feel restrictions or ease, and listen to the sound of the breath leaving your lungs. Notice its length. Continue to let your breath be natural without trying to change it in any way. It will usually begin to lengthen and become deeper as you relax and bring attention to it. Repeat this awareness practice with your hands resting on your lower ribs and finally again with your hands on your chest. Take note of movement, discomfort, restriction, sound, and length in each segment of the torso. Lastly, notice the spaces between inhalation and exhalation. Do you tend to hold your breath in or out? How does it feel when you are full of breath and also when the lungs are empty?

When I began my own yoga practice, my breath was so restricted and imbalanced between my left and right, back and front. Knowing that, I began to attend to my breath throughout the day a little more. Slowly, over time and with practiced attention, my breath pattern has completely changed and become more fluid, balanced, and full. The first step was paying attention.

PRANAYAMA

The meaning of the word *pranayama* has been debated for many years now. Broken down into its roots, *prana-yama* is often translated as "breath control" or "controlling life-force energy." It has also been broken down as *prana-ayama*, which is translated as the opposite, "liberation of breath" or "expansion of life-force energy." As a teacher and student, I have found that first learning to control or manipulate the breath leads to its liberation. It's not either/or but both, control and expansion.

We begin with the basic form of *pranayama* used in *asana* practice, known as *ujayii*, the "victorious" or "uprising" breath. Take a few minutes either reclined or seated to connect with your natural flow of breath first. To begin *ujayii*, inhale through your nose and exhale through your mouth as if you are trying to fog up a mirror. The back of the throat slightly contracts, creating a sound like the ocean. Let the breath be long and full, not harsh or loud. After a few repetitions close your mouth so that you inhale and exhale through your nose, maintaining this sound as you slightly constrict the back of your throat. Allow yourself to explore this breath—let it be stronger, then softer.

Use *ujayii* while practicing *asana*. Let it be soft and slow, especially during the beginning and ending of your practice. As you move through various postures, you will notice that the *ujayii* breathing becomes stronger during challenging poses such as deep forward folds, twists, backbends, or hand balancing. The sound of the breath helps us keep attention on the balance between effort and ease, helps steady our focus, and prepares the body and nervous system for deeper practices.

Many different *pranayama* techniques are taught; it is a whole world of practice unto itself. For the purposes of this book, *ujayii* and *nadi shodhana*, "channel cleansing," are the most accessible with the greatest benefits for most athletes. *Nadi shodhana*, also known as "alternate nostril breathing," is said to be a purifying breath that has been shown to balance the left and right hemispheres of the brain as well as the sympathetic and parasympathetic nervous systems. Before we get into the practice itself, let's look at these systems and how they relate to stress.

As part of the autonomic nervous system, which is involuntary, the sympathetic nervous response kicks in when we perceive a threat. Known commonly as the "fight, flight, or freeze" response, it is triggered when we feel threatened and prepares the body for escape or defense. Quickly, a flood of hormones intensifies the senses and heart rate, sending extra blood to the muscles in preparation for flight or fight. The breath quickens, delivering fresh oxygen to the brain, and glucose is boosted into the bloodstream for quick energy. Digestive processes slow down or halt and muscles tense. Typically once the threat is faced or removed, most animals will shake to release this stored stress and the body resumes homeostasis. Shaking during shock is one of these responses. As the stress recedes, the parasympathetic response, also known as "rest and digest" mode, kicks in. Tension releases, the heart and respiratory rate slow, the digestive response resumes, and a flood of calming hormones kicks in. However, we can, and as modern humans often do, get stuck in this "fight, flight, or freeze" response. *Pranayama* and deep breathing practices help us restore balance between these systems.

Alternate nostril breathing, *nadi shodhana*, helps restore harmony between these systems and is very effective at turning on the parasympathetic response when

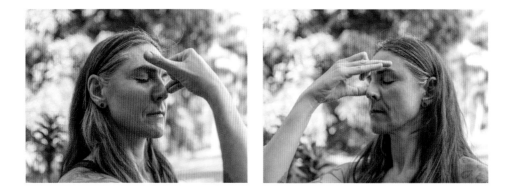

practiced regularly. Begin by consciously attuning to your breath in a seated posture. Practice *ujayii* for a few minutes to expand the breath. Using your dominant hand, place your thumb on one side of your nostrils and your ring finger on the opposite nostril. Use a light touch and hold this hand position without closing the nostrils as you take a few breaths. To begin, close the right nostril and inhale through the left. Then close the left side, release the right, and exhale through the right nostril. Inhale through the right side and then exhale through the left side. This completes one round of *nadi shodhana*. Repeat this for five to fifteen rounds, keeping your posture upright but relaxed. End with a few minutes of *ujayii* and then rest in your natural breath either seated or reclining in corpse pose.

This can be done at the end of your *asana* practice when your body is relaxed and you have created more space within. Some yoga lineages and teachers start with the right nostril, while others begin with the left. I have been taught to begin with the left side, so that is what is offered here. Feel free to play with this and discover what feels most calming and centering for you.

Begin by incorporating *ujayii* in your yoga practice. Once you feel comfortable, begin practicing *nadi shodhana* afterward. Start slowly with just five to eight rounds of alternate nostril breathing. Add more rounds when you feel ready, and please go at your own pace. I have found this breath practice very effective when I have had a stressful day or experience. Remember, stress is not a bad thing. We will always have stressors in life—this is how we grow and change. But staying in a chronic stress response is extremely deleterious to our overall health and well-being. Learn to release stress and get into "rest and digest" mode often. Outdoor athletes face stressors all the time in different forms. Practice these breathing techniques on and off the mat to support you in your adventurous life.

THE TAKEAWAY

We breathe all day and night, but most of us are not very conscious of our breathing patterns or how they affect our overall vitality. Our breath is the easiest and most accessible way to shift our mental and emotional states. Using the breathing awareness and expansion practices of yoga can have great benefits for our fitness, recovery, and emotional well-being.

- First become aware of your natural breathing patterns by using the short exercises listed earlier.

- Begin using *ujayii* breathing in your yoga practice and even in your sports.

- Start slowly with the practice of *nadi shodhana* until you get the hang of it. Then begin to do more repetitions, increasing over time.

- Yogic and deep breathing helps balance the nervous system and physiological responses of the body/mind very effectively.

- Be gentle and curious with the practices, and take them off the mat into your life.

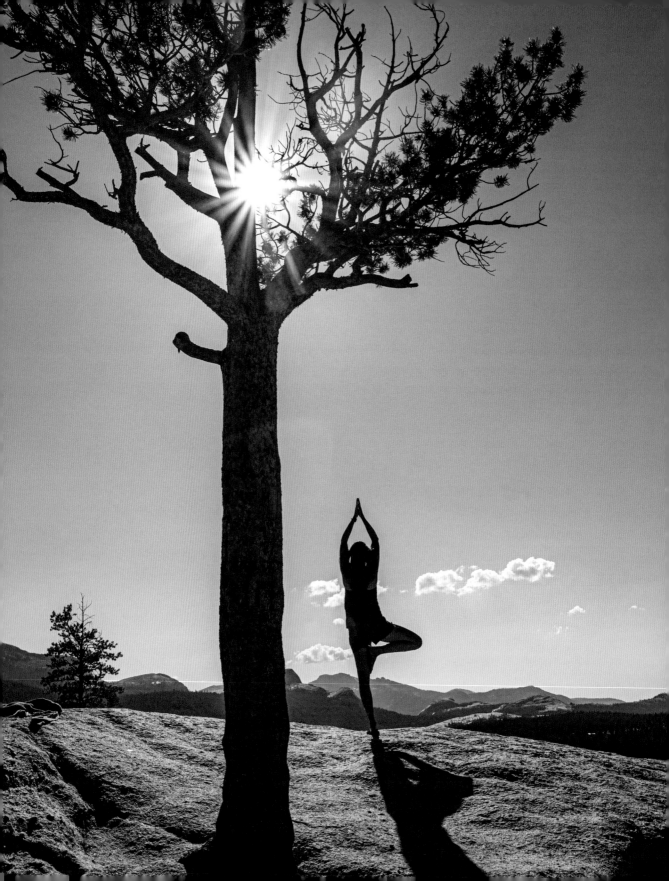

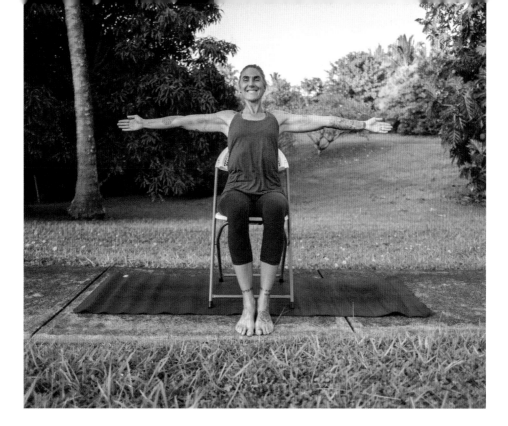

CHAPTER 5

ASANA

The body is the bow, asana is the arrow and the soul is the target.
B. K. IYENGAR

IT IS SAID THAT THE PRACTICE OF YOGA *asana* is a moving meditation. By balancing effort and surrender, paying close attention to our breath and each moment, we move deeper into a centered and calm state of being, not doing. But this, of course, takes practice and patience, as with learning anything. This chapter explains each posture that is used later in the sport-specific sequences. Instructions are included for getting into and out of each pose as you begin to practice as well as tips for adapting poses and possible risks to be mindful of. I suggest reading through all the poses and getting familiar with the basic shapes shown in the photographs. As you begin to practice sequences for your favorite sports, you can refer back to this chapter for detailed instructions and tips.

> **"** IN ADDITION, WITH PROPER *UJAYII* BREATHING AND ALIGNMENT, THE DEEP ABDOMINAL AND SPINAL MUSCLES ARE ENGAGED THROUGHOUT THE PRACTICE OF YOGA."

Pose Notes

Sanskrit: For the purposes of this book and for greater accessibility, I use the common English name of each posture. Due to the different names used for postures among different yoga lineages, I also include the Sanskrit names most commonly used, when available. Modern yoga has evolved so much over the years that there are some postures that do not have traditional Sanskrit names.

Tips: At the end of most of the descriptions for the postures are tips for practicing the pose in a way that makes it more accessible, deepens the pose, or offers a secondary variation.

Adaptive postures: Many postures can be done while sitting in a chair or wheelchair or while lying down. When possible, adapted versions are offered based on sitting in a chair. The sit bones are the foundation of chair variations. Sit tall and root evenly through both sides of your seat, adjusting to find a neutral pelvis before you begin. Some types of postures, such as inversions and hand balancing poses, are not easily adapted. For the purposes of this book, I have included images for the poses most easily accessible from a chair. Many postures done lying down on the back or belly are accessible as well.

Possible risks: At the end of each description for the postures is a list of areas of the body that could be at risk with the pose. For instance, if you already have knee pain, a shoulder injury, or low back injury, you will want to use caution when practicing a pose that puts pressure on that particular area. This may mean taking an easier variation, not staying in the pose as long, or even skipping the pose until you recover or build the needed strength and mobility to practice it safely.

WARMING UP

As with any physical exercise or movement practice, it is important to warm up the whole body. Moving blood, lymph, and synovial fluid throughout the body will prepare your muscles, tendons, ligaments, and joints for whatever activity you are about to do. It helps work out the kinks, bring more balance to our sides and deep spinal muscles as well as increasing the range of motion of joints. It also begins the expansion of the breath and increases cardiovascular health. Depending on your sport(s) of choice, you will want to target specific areas that will be stressed such as your hands and forearms if you are a climber. Snowboarders and skiers will want to spend more time on the lower body and core. Specific sequences of postures for each sport are listed in the sport-specific chapters in this book. Take some time to familiarize yourself with the *asanas* and instructions in this section and then refer back to it as you develop your practices.

Joint Rotations

Rotating all your major joints is a great way to relieve stiffness, improve blood flow, and awaken the mind-body connection gently. It can be done anywhere and is especially helpful after you have been sitting for long periods while working or driving to your adventure destination. Repeat rotations eight to fifteen times in each direction while breathing deeply and paying attention to the sensations.

NECK

Circle your head one direction, leading with your nose and keeping some extension through the crown of your head. Repeat in the other direction. If you experience pain, make your circles smaller or do half circles.

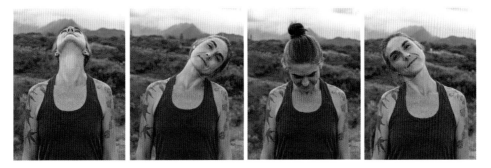

SHOULDERS

Keeping your neck and head neutral, lift your shoulders up to your ears, then back, down, and forward in a circular motion, continuing through your repetitions. Repeat in the opposite direction.

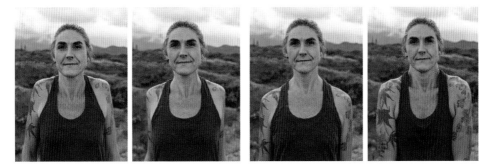

WRISTS

Holding your arms out in front of you at shoulder height, circle your wrists twelve to twenty times in each direction.

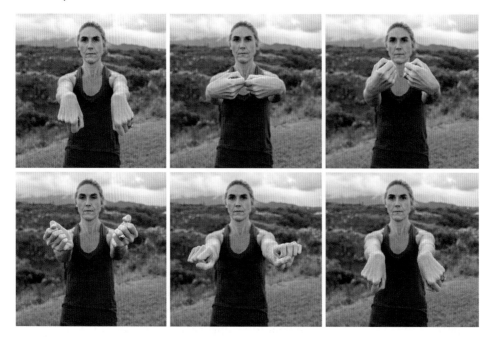

HIPS

With your hands on your hips, circle your hips around in one direction as if you are hula hooping. Repeat in the other direction, making your circles as big as you can. Aim to keep your torso upright and feet grounded as you do this.

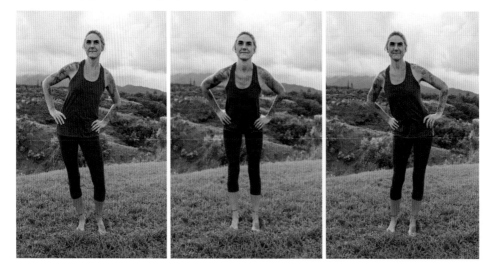

KNEES

Bend over at the hips, place your hands on your knees, and bend the knees a bit. Circle the knees in one direction eight to fifteen times, then go the other way. Make your circles as big as you can without pain.

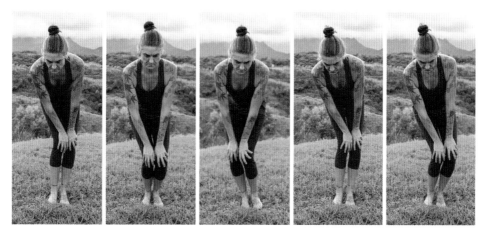

ANKLES

While standing on one foot, lift the other leg up, bending at the knee. Rotate the lifted ankle in one direction eight to fifteen times, then go the other direction. Repeat on the second side. Keep your torso upright and gaze forward, holding onto a wall, counter, or chair back if you need help with balancing.

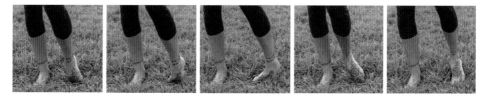

SPINAL ROLLS

Standing tall with feet hip distance apart, begin by dropping your chin to your chest and slowly roll downward, keeping your knees bent. Then roll back up the spine, one vertebrae at a time until you come to standing tall. This slow articulation of the spine helps to improve mobility, strength, and midline awareness.

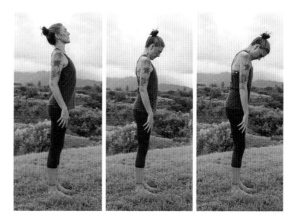

Reclined Warm Ups

These reclined warm ups are a great way to begin practice after long days and miles of hiking, snowboarding, skiing, or backpacking. They can be done on a mat, sleeping pad, bed, or wherever you can lie down. Start by lying on your back with your knees bent and feet on the ground hip distance apart in an active recovery pose.

RECLINED CENTERING POSE

This is often called active recovery pose and is the beginning setup for future postures. Start in a reclined position with your knees bent and feet on the ground. Let your whole body relax and breathe deeply for 3 to 5 minutes. Your arms can be by your side with the palms facing upward, or you can rest your hands on your belly.

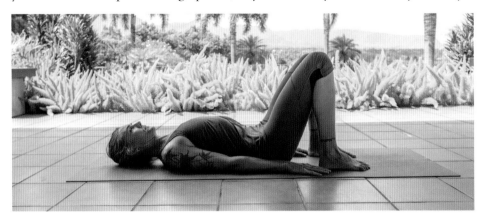

RECLINED KNEES TO CHEST POSE

Hug both of your knees toward your chest, either holding onto the backs of the legs or the front of the shins. Rock gently side to side and then back and forth along the spine if it feels good on your back. Stay for ten breaths or so.

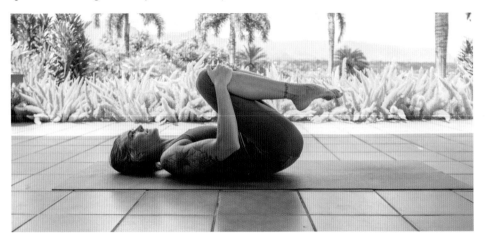

WIND RELIEVING POSE

From a reclined position bring one knee into your chest as far as you can, holding onto the back of the leg or the shin. Extend the other leg out along the ground, actively engaging all the muscles and rooting the heel, calf, and hamstrings down. Hug the bent knee into your chest, and on an exhalation take your chin to your chest, lifting your shoulders off the ground and reaching your forehead toward the knee. Stay for three to five breaths and then repeat on the second side. This pose lengthens the back muscles on one side while lengthening the iliopsoas and hip flexors on the extended leg. It also helps activate the hamstrings and glutes on the straight leg.

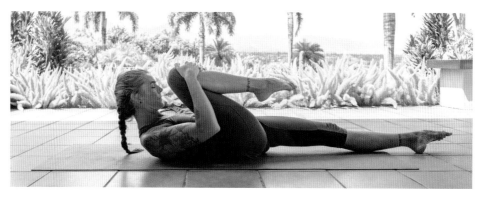

WINDSHIELD WIPER POSE

Starting in the active recovery pose, place your feet a little wider than hip distance apart. Take your arms out wide into a "T" position, pressing your palms down. Keeping the feet on the floor, drop your knees to the right on an exhalation, then come back to center on an inhalation. Drop the knees to the left on an exhalation and then return to center on an inhalation. Repeat five to eight times, then return to center. This is a good way to begin to warm up the low back, hips, and legs by internally and externally rotating the legs as you twist gently side to side. It can also help relieve stiffness in the low back.

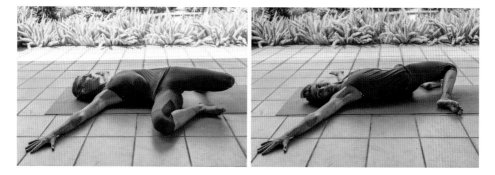

RECLINED TWIST

From active recovery pose, hug the right knee toward the chest, keeping the left leg extended on the ground. Take your right knee to the left, lying on the outside of the left leg. Take the knee down only as far as it goes comfortably. If the knees are hovering above the ground quite a bit, use a block or folded blanket under the knees for support. Take five to eight breaths, then repeat on the left side. This posture gently twists the spine, lengthening the back muscles and opening the chest on the opposite side.

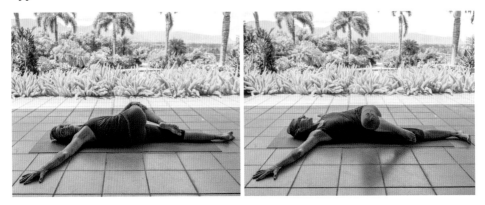

BRIDGE PRESS

From active recovery pose, bend your elbows to a 90-degree angle, pressing your arms down into the ground. Draw your shoulders close to the spine, rooting them into the ground. Press your feet down firmly and lift your hips up toward the sky, keeping your knees from splaying out. On an inhalation return to the starting position with a neutral low back. As you exhale, lift your hips toward the sky. Repeat with the breath pattern eight to fifteen times. This activates the shoulders, opens the chest, stretches the diaphragm, and engages the glutes and hamstrings. Lengthening the hip flexors and thigh muscles also helps prepare the body for sun salutations and more-active standing postures and backbends.

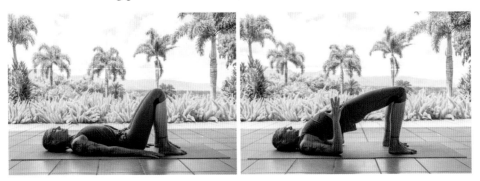

RECLINED FULL EXTENSION

Starting in active recovery pose, extend your legs out long on the floor, reaching through your heels and pressing your legs and hips firmly down into the ground. Extend your arms overhead alongside your ears, reaching through your fingers and pressing your shoulders downward. Keep your head in a neutral position, gazing upward. Take eight to ten long breaths, lengthening the whole body and rooting downward into the earth to open up the front body. Eventually, when you come up to standing you will have this imprint in your body memory to help you stabilize your low back and front ribs.

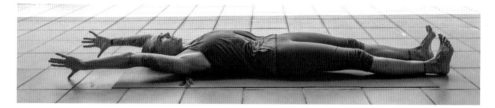

Dynamic Warm Ups

CHILD'S POSE

The classical form of child's pose has the knees together, forehead on the floor, and the arms draped at your sides with the hands down by the hips. Begin with your shins on the ground, knees together. From there lengthen your spine forward, placing your forehead on the mat or a block. Let your arms drape at your sides. Stay for five to ten breaths, letting the pelvis ground, thighs lengthen, ankles stretch, and back release.

A variation of child's pose takes the knees apart, allowing more room for the torso to fold forward. The arms are stretched forward with the hands actively pressing into the ground to settle the hips back and open the chest. If your forehead doesn't reach the ground, place a block under it. Stay for five to ten breaths.

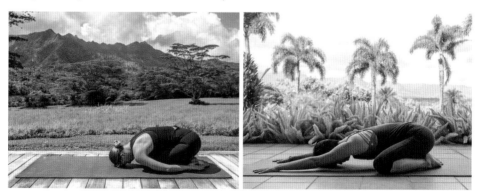

CAT AND COW POSES

Cat pose, also known as *marjaryasana*, stretches the back, hips, and wrists as well as engages the core. Find table pose to begin: on your hands and knees with your hands shoulder width apart, fingers spread and rooting. The knees are hip distance apart and directly under the hips. Press your shins and the tops of your feet down firmly. From table pose tilt your pelvis back, lifting your belly up and rounding your chin toward your chest. Your spine rounds toward the sky just as a scared cat does. Stay for a few breaths.

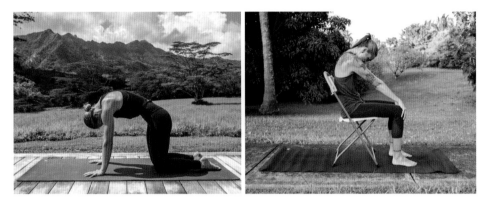

Cow pose, *bitilisana*, stretches the front of the body and wrists while opening the top chest as the back and shoulder muscles all engage. The inner thighs and groins move back and apart, increasing the curve in the low back. From table pose tilt your pelvis forward, lengthen the abdomen, and reach your chest forward as the chin lifts upward. Press your hands and shins down firmly. Stay for a few breaths. Alternating between cat and cow pose with the breath helps activate all the muscles of the core and shoulders while also lengthening them. The spine moves through flexion and extension, waking up the abdominal muscles and also stretching open the chest, expanding the lungs. Move slowly as you breathe, and repeat the movements five to ten times each.

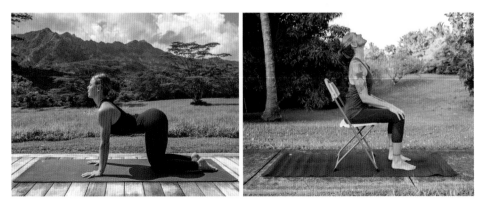

TWISTING TABLE POSE

This pose (sometimes referred to as thread-the-needle) begins to loosen up the muscles along the back and shoulders while creating a gentle twist for the spine. Begin in table pose, rooting down through the hands and shins and keeping the head extending forward. Lift your right arm out to the side and upward, following with your gaze as you open into a twist. Then take the right arm under the body, threading it toward the left of your mat. Rest your right shoulder and head on the ground with your right palm facing up. Look up toward the sky and root your knees into the earth as you breathe into your back. Stay for five breaths or so and repeat on the second side.

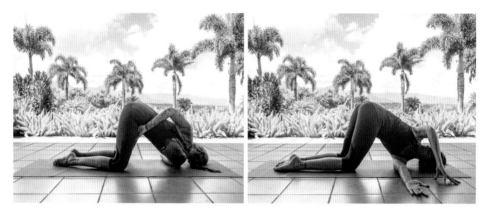

FIRE HYDRANT POSE

While cat and cow pose engage the extensors and flexors of the hips, this pose engages the lateral rotators, which help stabilize the pelvis. Begin in table pose with your head extended, hands and shins grounding. Lift your right knee up and out to the side, engaging the side of the hip and keeping the rest of your body as stable as possible. Hold for five breaths, or lift and lower back to table, repeating five to ten repetitions. Repeat on the left leg.

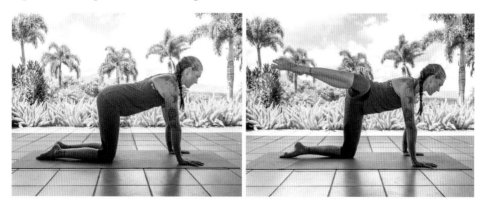

PUPPY POSE

While not a classical pose, this stretch helps prepare the body for downward facing dog pose by opening up the chest while stabilizing and stretching the shoulders and back. Start in table pose, then walk your hands forward as far as you can while keeping your hips above your knees. Either the toes can be tucked under or the tops of the feet can be grounded. Lengthen your abdomen and stretch through your arms as you breathe. Take your groins and inner thighs back and apart as you lift the belly and lengthen. Stay for five to ten breaths.

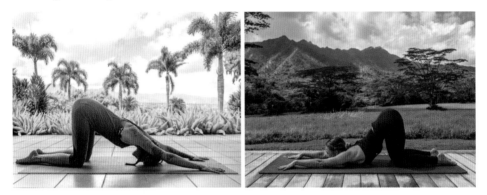

DOWNWARD FACING DOG

Adho mukha svanasana, otherwise known as downward facing dog or down dog pose, is a common foundation posture that is part of the sun salutation and vinyasa flow practices. It is a semi-inversion, meaning the pelvis is above the heart and head. It stretches the chest, shoulders, abdomen, back, glutes, and back of the legs while strengthening the shoulder girdle. Begin in table pose, pressing the fingertips down firmly and straightening the arms, keeping your head extended. Tuck your toes under and lift your knees off the ground, stretching your sit bones back. Root through your hands and extend from your shoulders back down into the earth. Lift your belly up and back. Stay for five to ten breaths.

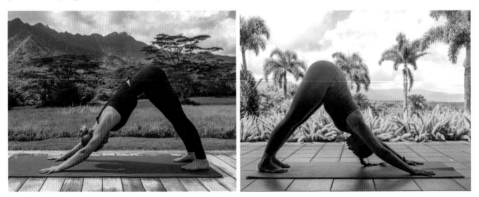

If your calves and hamstrings are feeling tight, bend one knee at a time, walking the legs out a bit to warm up the muscles until you can stay steady in the pose. For beginners and those with low back pain or injury, feel free to keep your knees bent a little whenever you take this pose.

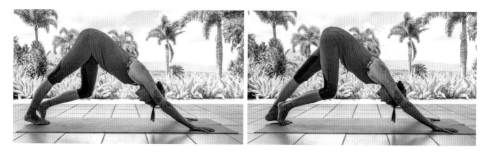

HIGH PLANK AND FOUR LIMBED STAFF POSE

This pair of postures is excellent for building core and postural strength. *Chaturanga dandasana* also strengthens the legs, hips, shoulders, and arms. Begin in table pose on hands and knees with your hands shoulder width apart and knees under the hips. Lengthen your spine, bringing your belly up and in, and press your hands down firmly to engage the chest and shoulders. Keeping the neck long and head neutral, tuck your toes under and on an exhalation lift your knees and straighten your legs, coming up into high plank, also known as top of a push-up. Hold the plank with arms straight for five to ten breaths as you widen through the shoulders and press back through your heels, keeping your core engaged. To lower into full *chaturanga dandasana*, bend your elbows, drawing them back toward your hips as you move forward onto your toes. Keep your crown extending forward and your core engaged as you hold this position with your elbows bent at 90 degrees or so. Take three to five breaths before either returning to high plank or lowering the knees and moving back into child's pose.

Tips: Try placing a block between your thighs as you practice this pose. Squeeze the block, engaging your inner thighs, outer hips, and lower belly. Stay as long as you can, breathing deeply. To build the strength for this pose, try starting from a half plank with the knees down.

Possible risks: Low back, shoulders, and wrists.

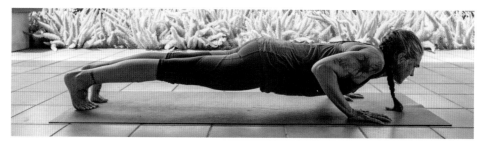

ALTERNATING LOCUST POSE

Locust pose is a gentle backbend and a fundamental posture for strengthening the muscles of the back of the body and lengthening the front body. I like to do this pose in my warm ups to counteract sitting and modern life. From table pose, lie on your belly with your arms extended in front of you and legs stretching back along the floor. Turn your palms to face each other so your thumbs are up and pinky fingers are down. Hug your legs toward the midline and lengthen as you inhale. Lift and press your head back to initiate spinal extension, then lift and extend your right arm and left leg, keeping both as straight as you can. Relax to the ground on an inhalation. Repeat on the other side, lifting the left arm and right leg on an exhalation. Continue alternating sides as you breathe for ten to twenty rounds. This activates a cross body connection and prepares the body for deeper back extension postures.

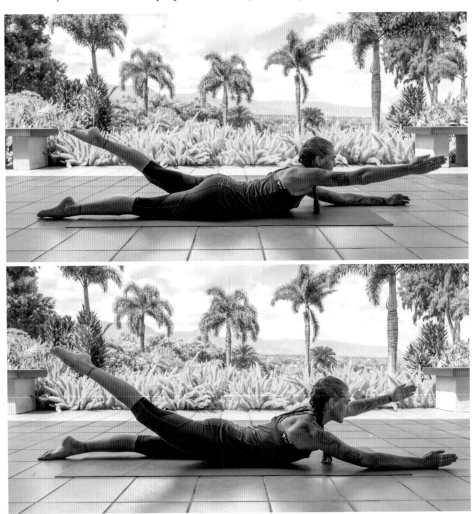

COBRA POSE

Bhujangasana, cobra posture, extends the front of the body, lengthening the hip flexors, abdominal muscles, and chest even more than locust pose. It strengthens the shoulders, low back, hips, and legs as well. This is a wonderful pose for relieving back pain and restoring balance to your posture after long days adventuring. Begin by lying on your belly with your legs extending long and your hands on either side of your chest. Pressing your fingers, pelvis, and legs down firmly, inhale and lengthen the belly and chest forward. As you exhale, move your head and chest forward and up away from the floor, engaging your shoulder blades toward the spine and down the back. Isometrically pull back on your hands to further engage the back of the shoulders, and actively extend your legs back and down. Stay for five to eight breaths and release back down to the floor.

Tips: When you become comfortable with the posture, you may begin to work deeper by placing the hands closer to your lower ribs and lifting more of the front body off the ground.

Possible risks: Low back, shoulders, wrists, and neck.

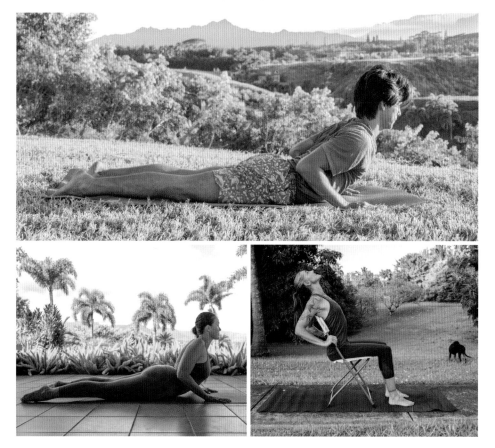

UPWARD FACING DOG POSE

This posture builds on the foundation of mobility and strength from locust, cobra, and downward facing dog poses. Upward facing dog pose, *urdhva mukha svanasana*, is a deeper backbend and spinal extension that builds strength in the back of the body and greater length in the front of the body. Begin as for cobra, with your legs extended and the tops of the feet firmly rooting into the ground. Place your hands as close down by your hips as you can, with the palms flat, fingers spread and pressing firmly. Inhaling, lengthen the back of your neck while looking straight down at the ground, fully engage your entire body, and squeeze your shoulders onto your back toward your spine. Exhaling, push your hands down and draw the chest forward as you lift your legs, pelvis, and torso off the ground until your arms and legs are straight. Draw your shoulders back and lift your belly, drawing the floating ribs inward as you reach powerfully back through your legs. Stay for three to five breaths before either coming down to the ground to rest or moving back into downward facing dog pose.
Tips: Try practicing this pose with your hands on blocks to create more space for the spine to lengthen and the pelvis to extend. Keep your legs actively extending.
Possible risks: Low back, shoulders, wrists, and neck.

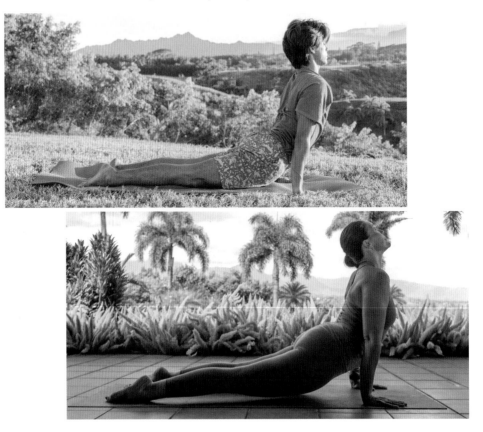

STANDING POSES

MOUNTAIN POSE

Mountain pose, *tadasana* or *samshitthi*, is essentially anatomical neutral. However, the stresses of modern human life and adventure sports may make this posture challenging. The whole body is both slightly engaged and relaxed as we stand tall and strong. Come to standing with your feet hip distance apart. Spread your toes and ground your feet from the inner to outer edges, balancing the weight evenly. Root down through your feet, engaging your lower legs, thighs, hamstrings, and glutes a little. Your pelvis should be neutral (pubic bone in the same vertical plane as the ASIS). Lift up through the low belly and lengthen the torso on all sides as you gently draw your shoulders back and down. Extend up through the crown of your head so your eyes and chin are level. Stretch down through your fingertips. The palms may face in toward the thighs or be turned forward with fingers spread wide. Pressing palms together at heart center is a common variation that draws energy and attention to the centerline. Standing tall and rooting down, feel your center of gravity in the pelvis. Stay alert and relaxed as you take five to ten breaths.

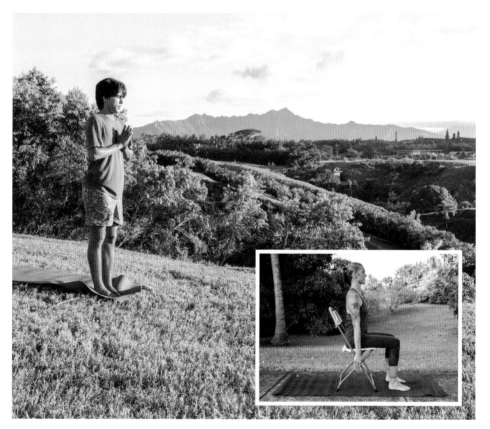

UPWARD SALUTE POSE

Urdhva hastasana, upward salute, is a common way to lengthen and engage the whole body by extending upward against gravity. It is also the beginning of the sun salutation sequence. From mountain pose, lift your arms overhead as you root evenly through your feet. Depending on the mobility of your shoulder girdle and tension in the hips, your arms may stay slightly in front of the head or extend just behind the ears. Aim to maintain a neutral pelvis by lifting the belly and breathing into the back of the lungs. Draw your front ribs in and down slightly, even if this brings your arms forward a bit. Take five to eight breaths here before releasing back to mountain pose.

Tips: Try doing this posture with your back at a wall or tree in order to feel the support of the back body and increase your spatial awareness. Keep most of your back body, hips, ribs, shoulders, and head against the wall or tree to improve your spinal alignment. Then translate this awareness to the posture away from the wall.

Possible risks: Low back and neck.

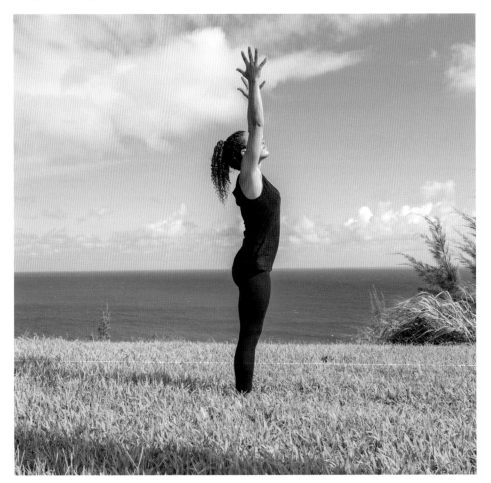

STANDING CRESCENT POSE

This posture is a beginning side stretch and helps lengthen the side body and strengthen spinal muscles. Begin in upward salute with your arms extended fully and clasp your hands together. Rooting down through both feet and keeping a neutral pelvis, extend your upper body on an exhalation toward the right to lengthen the left side. Look past your left arm to open the chest more. Stay for five breaths, then return to center on an inhalation and repeat the posture extending toward the left side. Keep both feet rooting and the pelvis facing forward, and actively contract the side you are leaning toward as you lift and lengthen the opposite side. Return to mountain pose when complete.

Tips: To help engage your legs and core in this pose, place a block between the thighs and squeeze. This helps activate the inner thighs, outer hips, and lower abdominal muscles.

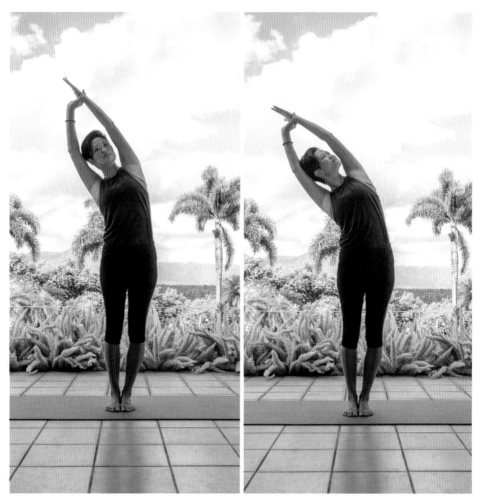

CHAIR POSE

This pose, *utkatasana*, activates the largest muscles and improves thigh strength, lower body mobility, and upper body alignment. It is a great way to prepare the body for standing poses. Beginning in mountain pose, reach your arms out in front of you as you sit your hips back and down as if you were about to sit on a chair. Bend your knees and ankles deeply and lift up through your torso, extending your spine. Taking the arms overhead as in upward salute increases the challenge to the back muscles. If you do take your arms overhead, extend fully and draw your belly up and back and your front ribs down slightly to even the curves in the spine. Take five or more breaths here before releasing into mountain pose.

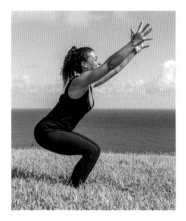

Tips: Practice this posture with a chair behind you a few times to get the feel of deeply sitting back into the hips. Another way to work with this posture is with a strap or bandana between your hands. Pull wide against the strap or bandana to help engage the shoulders and upper back as you move in and out of the pose a few times. Then translate without a strap.

Possible risks: Knees, low back, and shoulders.

STANDING FORWARD FOLD POSE

Uttanasana, standing forward fold, is a foundational posture that is also part of sun salutations and the vinyasa style of practice. Beginning in mountain pose, bring your hands to your hips, lengthen the front of the body, and hinge forward from the hips. Continue lengthening the front body as you bend forward. Once you have gotten to your first stopping point, bring your hands to either blocks or the ground. As you breathe here, root your feet downward and lift your hips upward. Fold deeper as you

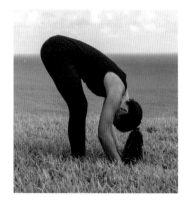

exhale, engaging the core and front of the legs. The entire back of the body is stretching from the calves all the way to the base of the skull. As you begin this posture, feel free to bend your knees as much as you need to and use blocks under the hands for support. Stay for five to eight breaths, letting your head and neck release.

Tips: Practice this pose facing a wall so that you can lean your upper back into the support and work the balance point more toward the center or front of your feet instead of the heels. Let your head and neck release as you stay for ten breaths.

Possible risks: Hamstrings and low back.

LOW LUNGE POSE

Anjaneyasana, low lunge, is also part of the sun salutation series and is an excellent posture for lengthening the hip flexors and the upper body. It also places the front ankle into deep flexion, preparing it for later postures. From forward fold, step the left foot back, bringing the knee down to the ground. If putting pressure on your kneecap is painful, place a thin blanket under the knee for padding. Bring your hands onto your front thigh, lifting your torso upright. Pressing your right foot and left knee downward, let your pelvis move forward and downward toward the ground. Keep your legs engaged and your low belly lifting. Either bring the hands to the hips or extend the arms to the sky as you extend the spine upward. Take five to eight deep breaths here, staying engaged. Step forward to *uttanasana*, then step the right foot back to repeat on the second side.

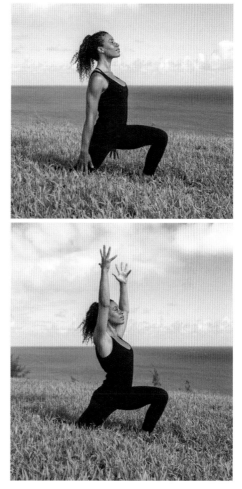

Tips: Begin this pose with your back thigh perpendicular to the ground to find a neutral pelvic tilt. Maintain a neutral pelvis as long as possible as you move deeper into the pose. It is easy to dump the pelvis forward and overarch the low back due to hip flexor tension or lack of lower abdominal strength. Hug your back knee and front foot toward each other to engage the legs fully.

Possible risks: Knees and low back.

CRESCENT LUNGE POSE

This pose, *ashta chandrasana*, is a more accessible variation of warrior one pose. It is excellent for beginners and people with low back pain or sacroiliac dysfunction because it keeps the pelvis squared forward and lengthens the hip flexors. Beginning in forward fold, step your left foot back, keeping the knee lifted off the ground and toes tucked under. Bring your hands to your front thigh as you bend your right knee toward a 90-degree angle or so. Root through your right foot; lift your torso upward, engaging through your core and back; and extend through the back leg, lifting your thigh upward. The hands can stay on the hips as you breathe, or you can extend your arms toward the sky. Stay for five to eight breaths, and then step forward and repeat on the second side.

Tips: Feel free to keep the back knee bent slightly to maintain a more neutral pelvis. As you work with this pose and other postures, the hip flexors will lengthen and the back leg may eventually be straighter. Also, shifting your weight forward into the front foot and lifting onto the toes of the back foot can help make more space in the low back by decreasing tension on the back leg's hip flexors.

Possible risks: Hips and low back.

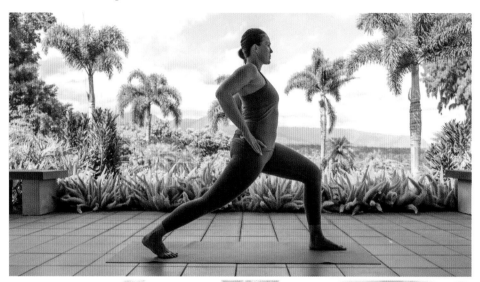

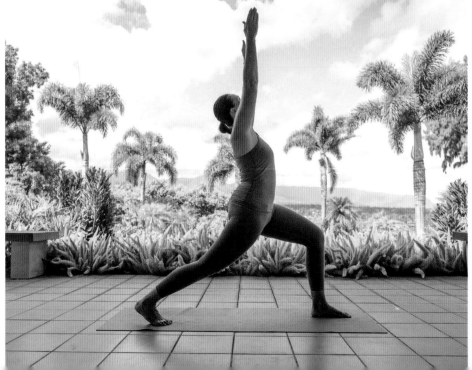

WARRIOR ONE POSE

Once you have gotten comfortable with crescent lunge pose, begin to work toward warrior one pose, *virabhadrasana one*. This is a deeper posture that requires more mobility in the hips and the ankle of the back leg. From forward fold, step the left foot back and turn the foot out slightly to ground the back heel down. Rooting through both feet, lift your torso upward and extend your arms to the sky, spreading your fingers. Like crescent pose, the back leg extends strongly, the belly lifts up and back, and the back muscles engage to lift the spine and extend the arms. Gaze upward slightly and stay for five to eight breaths. Step forward to fold, then step the right foot back, repeating on the second side.

Tips: This is a challenging pose for the low back. Try taking a shorter stance front to back and widening the feet apart left to right to create more space to turn the pelvis forward.

Possible risks: Knees, low back, shoulders, and neck.

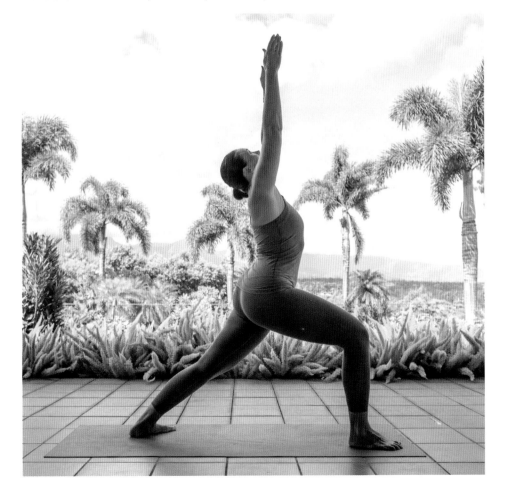

Sun Salutations

Surya namaskar, sun salutations, are a series of postures linked together through the breath that warm up the whole body. They can be done after the above warm ups toward the end of a more gentle or short practice, or they can be done to prepare for standing postures, backbends, forward folds, hip opening, twists, and inversions. Many yogis use this series as their primary warm up or do five to ten rounds before their other, deeper postures. This is a description of the classical sun salutation sequence with breath instruction. If this is new to you, take your time getting comfortable with the breathing pattern and depth of postures. It is a lifelong practice.

SUN SALUTATION A

(1) Begin in mountain pose.

(2) Inhale to upward salute.

(3) Exhale to forward fold.

(4) Inhale to half forward fold by bringing the hands to the shins and lifting the torso to parallel with the floor.

(3) Exhale to forward fold.

(5) Step the left foot back to low lunge on an inhalation.

(6) Step back to plank pose on an exhalation.

(7) Move into cobra pose or upward facing dog on an inhalation.

(8) Move back to downward facing dog on an exhalation.

(9) Step the left foot forward to low lunge on an inhalation.

(10) Step forward and fold to forward bend on an exhalation.

(11) Inhale to half forward fold by bringing the hands to the shins and lifting the torso to parallel with the floor.

(12) Exhale to forward fold.

(13) Inhale to upward salute.

(14) Exhale back to mountain pose.

Repeat on the second side, leading with the right foot to complete one round of sun salutations.

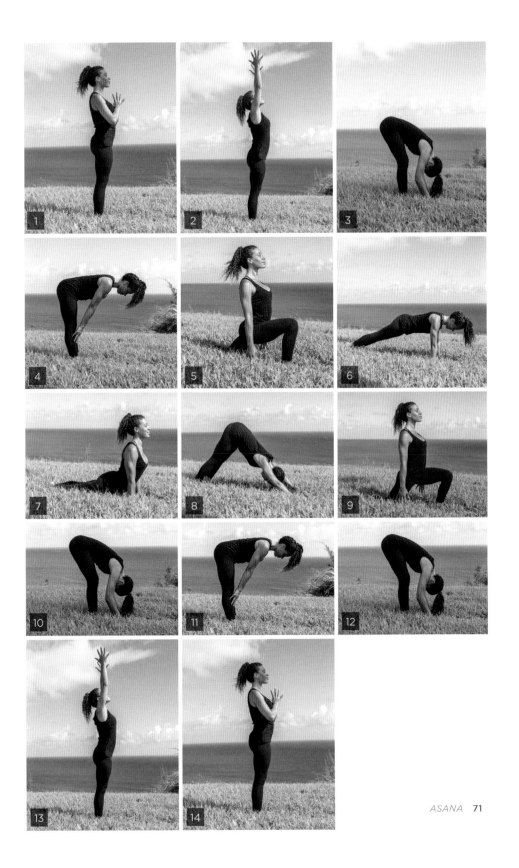

SUN SALUTATION B

Surya namaskar B is more challenging and can be done after five rounds of the classical sun salutation above. Typically five rounds are done before moving on to deeper postures.

- Take five full breaths in mountain pose.
- Inhaling, sit hips back in chair pose, lifting the arms to the sky.
- Exhale into forward fold.
- Step or hop back into high plank pose and exhale into four limbed staff pose.
- Inhale into cobra or upward facing dog pose.
- Exhale as you move into downward facing dog pose.
- Step your right foot forward between your hands, ground your back heel into the earth, and rise into warrior one pose for one breath.
- Step back into high plank and lower through four limbed staff pose on an exhale.
- Inhale into cobra or upward facing dog.
- Exhale into downward facing dog.
- Step the left foot forward between your hands, ground your back heel into the earth, and rise up into warrior one pose for a breath.
- Step back into high plank and lower through four limbed staff pose on an exhalation.
- Inhale into cobra or upward facing dog.
- Exhale into downward facing dog and stay for five breaths.
- Bend your knees, gaze forward, and either jump or step your feet forward toward the hands.
- Inhale to half forward fold by bringing the hands to the shins and lifting the torso to parallel with the floor.
- Exhale back into forward fold.
- Inhale, lifting into chair pose, arms extended toward the sky.
- Rooting down through your feet, inhale into upward salute.
- Exhale, bringing your hands to your heart. This concludes one round of sun salutation B.

EXTENDED SIDE ANGLE POSE

Utthita parsvakonasana, extended side angle pose, is another strong standing pose that engages and opens the legs, hips, torso, and shoulders while lengthening the side body. It is a foundational posture that prepares the body for deeper poses. From standing forward fold, step the left foot back, opening the hips and turning the toes so the outer edge of the foot is parallel with the back edge of your mat and the heel is grounded. Bend the right knee deeply and bring the right elbow to the knee, extending your left arm overhead alongside the ear, creating a line from the left foot to the left hand. Rooting into your feet, externally rotate the right thigh and turn your torso to face the long edge of your mat as you gaze to the side or up under the left arm. To deepen the pose, once your right thigh is parallel to the floor, you may take your right hand down to a block or the floor on the outside of the right foot. Take five to eight breaths here, then step forward and repeat on the second side.

Tips: Keep your back foot grounded with your leg fully engaged even as you deepen the bend in your front hip. Work the twist at the waist to open the chest.

Possible risks: Knees, hamstrings, low back, and shoulders.

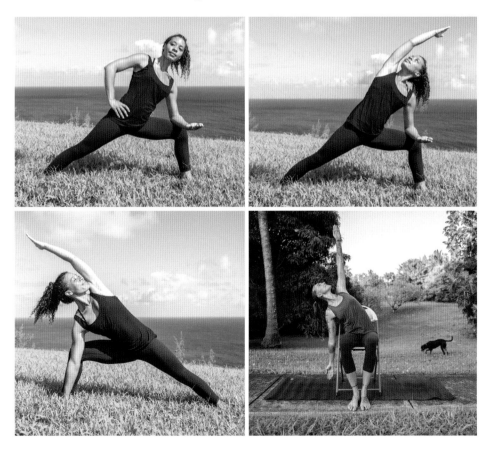

WARRIOR TWO POSE

Virabhadrasana two, warrior two pose, is a strong, energizing, and grounding posture that opens the chest and hips. From forward fold, step the left foot back and turn it out so the outer edge is parallel with the back edge of your mat. Bend the right knee directly over the toes. Grounding your feet, lift the torso up (perpendicular to the ground) and stretch your arms out to the sides. Your hips and chest will face the long edge of your mat in an open hip stance. The front thigh externally rotates while the back thigh internally rotates slightly. Bend the right knee as close to 90 degrees as you can, lift the low belly, and lengthen the torso upward, spreading your chest and shoulders wide apart as you gaze toward the tips of the fingers on the right hand. The tendency is to shift the torso forward, tipping at the pelvis and dropping the back arm. To balance this, reach outward through the back leg and arm, centering yourself. Stay for five to eight breaths, then step forward to forward fold and repeat on the second side.

Tips: First bring your shoulders directly over your hips. Draw your front ribs in and expand into the back of the body to bring greater balance to the pose.

Possible risk: Knees, low back, shoulders, and neck.

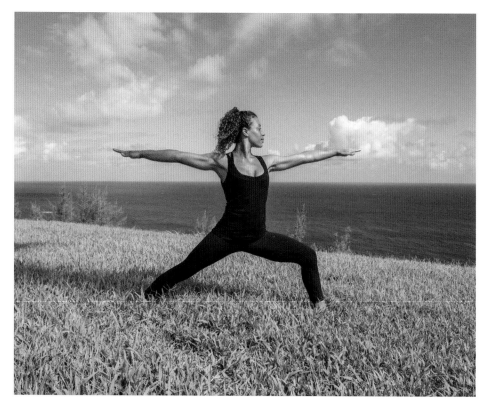

REVERSE WARRIOR POSE

This is a more modern posture that helps lengthen the front of the body and sides in preparation for deeper backbends. To enter *viparitta virabhadrasana two*, step into warrior two pose, then lift the front hand upward and the back hand softly down to the back hamstring. Maintain grounding the feet, engaging the legs with the front knee bent, and lifting the low belly and heart as you extend upward. Stay for five to eight breaths, then repeat on the other side after traditional warrior two.

Tips: Before entering this posture, shift your rib cage toward the back body and lift the lower belly. Then lean back to lengthen the front of the hips and torso, looking straight upward. Keep your back leg straight as you root down.

Possible risks: Knees, low back, shoulders, and neck.

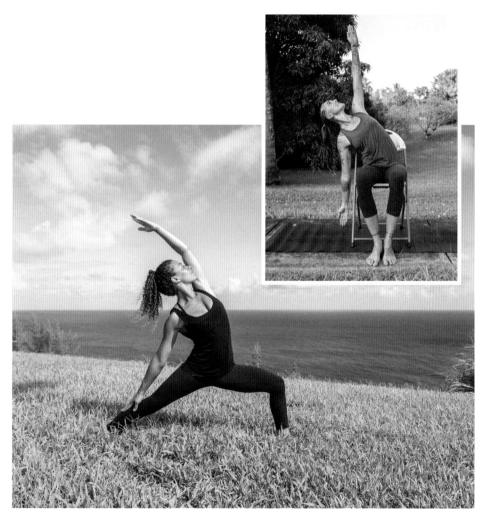

WARRIOR THREE POSE

This is a strong standing balancing pose that stabilizes the legs, core, and spine as you find steadiness. *Virabhadrasana three*, warrior three pose, helps increase single leg stability, which is key for hikers, backpackers, and climbers especially. From mountain pose, extend your arms overhead as you inhale. Extend your left leg up behind you as you bend forward at the hips. Keep your pelvis square toward the ground, engaging the low belly to keep a long spine. Arms can extend forward, or hands can press together in a prayer shape at your heart. Gaze may be down or toward the fingers (keeping the neck safe and long). Stay for five to eight breaths, then stand up and repeat on the second side.

Tips: If balance is hard for you, stand facing a wall and take the posture pressing your hands into the wall to help. You may also extend your arms along your sides toward your hips in the posture if extending the arms puts too much pressure on the shoulders.

Possible risks: Knees, hamstrings, and low back.

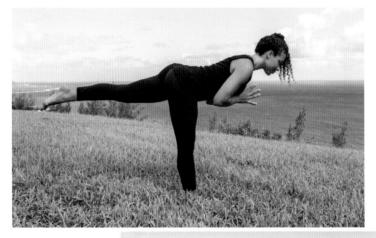

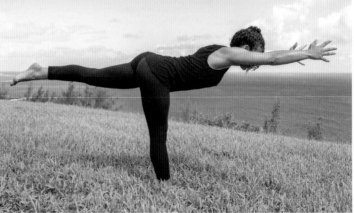

WIDE LEGGED FORWARD FOLD POSE

Prasarita padottanasana, wide legged forward fold, increases mobility in the ankles and hips while lengthening the inner thigh muscles, hamstrings, and back body. Stand in the center of your mat facing the long edge. Take your feet as wide apart as is comfortable, four feet or so, with your feet parallel. Bring your hands to your hips, inhale to lengthen the spine and lift the low belly, and hinge forward at the hips. Bend the knees as much as you need to, bringing your hands to the ground or to blocks. Lengthen the torso again on an inhale and fold deeply, bringing your hands farther back, maybe in line with the toes. Ground your feet and engage your legs and core while pressing your hands downward. Take five to eight breaths here and return to standing.

Tips: This posture may also be practiced against a wall to deepen the lengthening of the back muscles and hamstrings. Standing a foot or so facing a wall, bow forward into the posture, leaning your back against a wall with hands on the ground similar to *uttanasana*. As you get comfortable with this pose, you can try the different arm variations pictured below.

Possible risks: Knees, hamstrings, and low back.

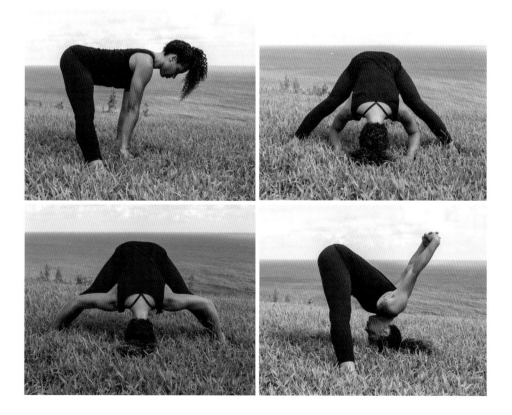

TRIANGLE POSE

Triangle pose, *utthita trikonasana*, is another strong standing posture that engages the legs, core, and back while lengthening the inner thighs and hamstrings. There is a gentle twist in the spine to open the torso and expand the chest. Standing at the top of your mat, step your left foot back 4 feet or so, turning your back foot out slightly to ground the heel and outer edge of the foot. With your right foot facing forward (to the top of the mat), straighten your right knee, engaging the whole leg. Inhale and extend both arms out to the side, widening the chest. Inhale and lift up through your torso and crown as you extend to the right, hinging at the hips. Keeping both feet grounded, bring your right hand to your shin, a block, or the floor and reach your left arm overhead. Turn your head so you can gaze toward the left hand, and extend through your crown, keeping your neck long. Take five to eight breaths here, then stand up and repeat on the second side.

Tips: The tendency here is to be passive through the front leg, round the spine toward the floor, or drop the head toward the ground. Rooting down through the front foot, externally rotating the thigh, will help turn the torso and support the spine and head. It is also helpful to practice this pose with your back against a wall to get the support to open fully.

Possible risks: Knees, hamstrings, low back, shoulders, and neck.

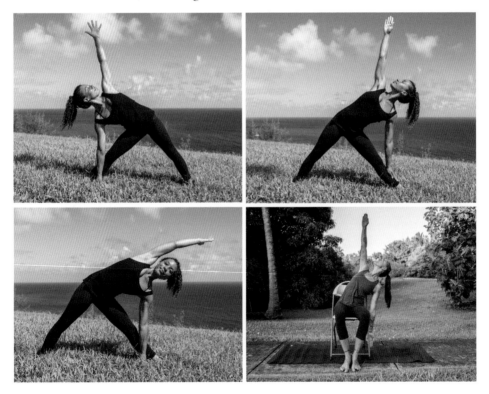

HALF MOON POSE

Ardha chandrasana, half moon pose, is an open hip pose similar to triangle, warrior two, and side angle pose. To enter the pose, begin in side angle pose with the right foot forward, left leg back. Bring the left hand to the left hip, reach the right hand forward a little, to the outside of the right foot, placing the fingers on the floor or hand on a block as you lift the left leg upward. Lift the left leg with the outer hip muscles, extending fully through the leg and foot. Turn the torso more open and extend the left arm toward the sky, turning the head to gaze at the hand. Stay for five to eight breaths, then return to side angle pose and repeat on the second side, entering from side angle.

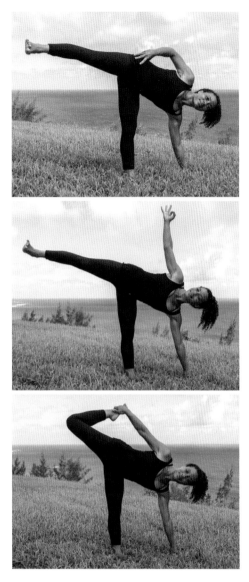

A variation of this pose that extends the hips and spine into more of a backbend is *ardha chandra chapasana*. From half moon pose with the left leg lifted, bend your left knee and reach the left hand back to take the foot or ankle. Kick the foot back into the hand and, rooting down into the right standing leg, press your hips forward and lengthen the spine back, opening up the hips and chest more. If you cannot take hold of your foot comfortably here, you can still bend the lifted knee and practice the opening, reaching your left hand back along your side. Stay for five breaths or so, release to half moon, then back to side angle pose. Stand up and repeat on the second side, entering through side angle.

Tips: This is another good posture to work at a wall. Have your back near a wall or solid surface so you can lean back into it and open the hips and chest more. If you are working with *chapasana* variation, give yourself a little more space from the wall to press your bound foot and hand into.

Possible risks: Knees, hamstrings, low back, shoulders, and neck.

PYRAMID POSE

Parsvottanasana, also known as pyramid pose, is a squared-hip posture that challenges balance; lengthens the spine, hamstrings, and calves; and increases mobility in the ankles and hips. From mountain pose, step the left foot back, only about 3 to 4 feet, keeping the hips facing forward. Turn the back foot out slightly to ground the back heel and the outer edge of the foot. Keep the width between the feet about hip distance. With your hands on your hips, lengthen your torso, hinging at the hips to extend forward. Bring your hands to blocks or the floor, keeping your back foot grounding, bending the front knee a little if needed. Continue to lengthen the spine and engage the legs as you take five to eight breaths. Bring your hands back to your hips and ground your feet to stand up out of the pose. Step forward and repeat on the second side.

Tips: This is a challenging posture. Try working with blocks under the hands and a wider stance left to right to find the squaring of the pelvis and rooting of the back foot. A traditional arm variation is to internally rotate the upper arms, bend the elbows, and bring the palms together behind the shoulders in reverse prayer position.

Possible risks: Knees, hamstrings, low back, and shoulders.

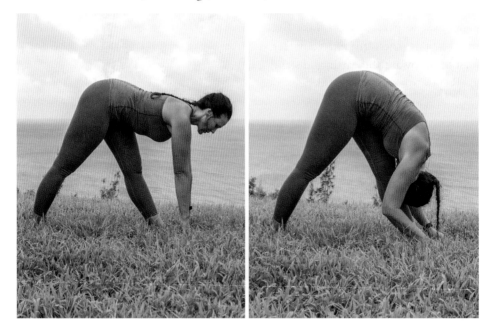

REVOLVED TRIANGLE POSE

Revolved triangle pose, *parivritta trikonasana*, is a squared-hip posture similar to pyramid pose but with a twist in the length of the spine and an opening across the chest. It is a challenging pose that strengthens the legs and core while lengthening the back body and spine. From pyramid pose with the left foot back, right foot forward, take the left hand to a block or the floor on the inside of the right foot. Keeping the feet grounded, lengthen your torso, extending through the crown, and twist toward the right. If this is very challenging for you, keep your right hand on your right hip. Otherwise, extend the right arm toward the sky, turning your head to gaze upward. Take five breaths or so, then ground your feet, turn back toward the earth, and stand up. Repeat on the second side, entering from pyramid pose.

Tips: Work with the lower hand on the inside of the front foot on a block for a while to get comfortable with the posture. Slowly, as you are ready, move the block closer to the inside of the front foot and then to the outside of the front foot. Then progress, if available, to removing the block and working with the hand down.

Possible risks: Knees, hamstrings, low back, shoulders, and neck.

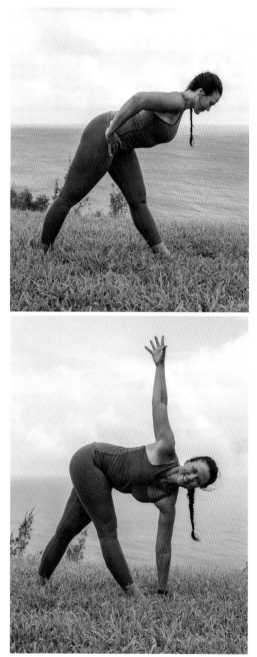

TREE POSE

Vrksasana, tree pose, is a great beginning balancing posture that strengthens the legs, core, and hips while elongating the inner thigh muscles. Balance poses in general help increase focus, inner stability, and static strength. Beginning in mountain pose, standing strong on your left foot, bend and turn the right knee out and lift your right foot up, placing it either on the inside of your left calf or thigh depending on your mobility. Press the foot into the leg and stabilize the left standing leg. Bring your hands to your heart in prayer pose. Rooting down, stand tall, keeping your front hip points facing forward as you externally rotate the right thigh bone. The hands can stay at the heart with the gaze forward, or you can extend your arms overhead reaching to the sky. Stay for five to ten breaths and repeat on the second side.

Tips: Practice this posture with your back against a wall or tree to find the alignment of the hips and spine. Then move away from the support as you get comfortable.

Possible risks: Knees, low back, and shoulders.

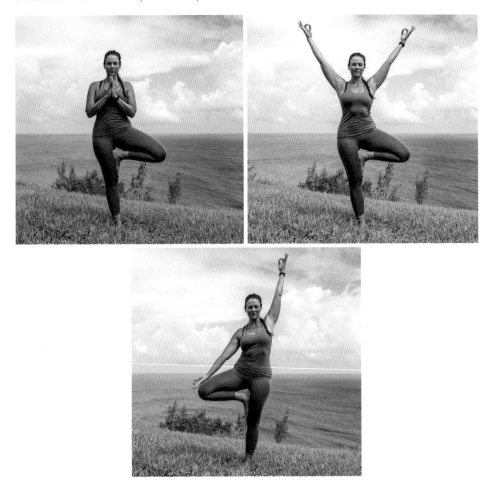

HAND TO BIG TOE POSE

Another grounding and centering balance posture is *utthita hasta padangusthasana*, hand to big toe pose. Like tree pose it strengthens the legs and pelvis; engages the core, arms, and shoulders; improves posture; and lengthens the hamstrings. Starting in mountain pose, ground into your left leg and foot. Bend your right knee, taking hold of your right big toe with your right hand. Stand tall, focusing your gaze forward, as you lift the right knee and foot up then extend the leg forward toward straight. It's better to bend the extended leg a little to keep your torso upright and shoulders engaged on the back. Stay for five to eight breaths, release, and repeat on the second side. A common variation of this posture takes the extended leg out to the same side while lifted. To do this, externally rotate the thigh bone as you take the leg out, lifting as much with your thigh and abdominal muscles as with the arm. Return to center and repeat on the second side after the first extension.

Tips: Using a strap to reach the bottom of the foot is a common modification. Working without a strap, though, and keeping the lifted leg bent, hand on the toes, is such a powerful way to work with this pose. It is humbling and honest, and teaches your body how to hold steady in your optimal spinal alignment.

Possible risks: Knees, hamstrings, low back, and shoulders.

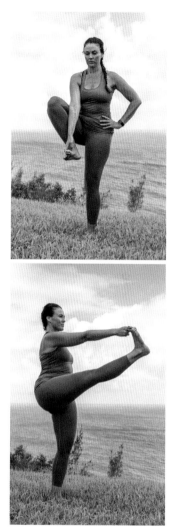

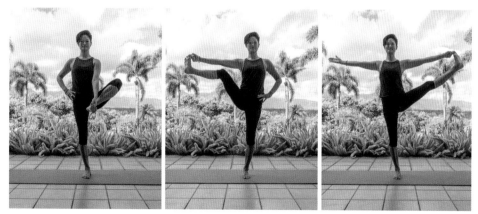

STANDING PIGEON POSE

This posture, *tada kapotasana*, is a preparation for a much more challenging hand balance pose and is excellent for targeting the lateral rotator muscles of the outer hips. It strengthens the legs and the core while lengthening the back muscles. Beginning in mountain pose, stand strong on your left foot and cross the right ankle over the left thigh above the knee. Sit back into chair pose from here, keeping your hips centered and facing forward with hands at the heart. As you bend the left knee and ankle more, the outer right hip will begin to stretch. Your hands may stay at your heart in prayer or rest on the right leg as you bend forward at the hips. Take five to eight breaths, then come to mountain pose and repeat on the second side.

Tips: Keep the foot that is crossed flexed and press the ankle down into the other thigh to increase the leverage and opening of the outer hip. Another way to practice with the pose is to fold forward, bringing your hands to blocks or the ground to deepen the posture.

Possible risks: Knees and low back.

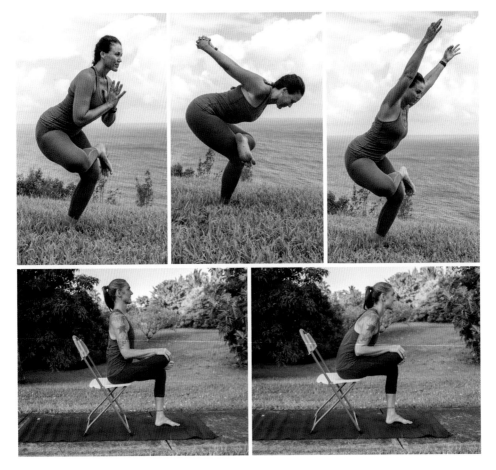

REVOLVED HAND TO BIG TOE POSE

This posture combines balance, twisting, and outer hip lengthening as well as chest opening. It helps warm up the whole body, focus the mind, and improve posture as you move on to other poses in your practice. *Parivritta hasta padangusthasana*, revolved hand to big toe pose, builds from the foundation of hand to big toe pose and revolved triangle pose. Begin by standing tall with your weight shifted to your left foot. Bring your right knee up to hip height, holding on with both hands. Maintain the strength and balance on your left foot as you begin to twist toward your right. Bring your right hand to your right hip as you deepen the twist, or extend your arm out straight, reaching through the right fingertips. Stay for three to five breaths before returning to center and repeating on the second side. One variation of this posture is to hold onto the big toe and extend the lifted leg out straight as you twist toward it.

Tips: Rooting through your standing leg and pressing the thigh back slightly will help you maintain your balance and posture as you twist. All variations of this posture can be done against a wall for support and also to deepen the twist. Just stand a few inches away from the wall to give yourself space to twist and press your hands into the wall for leverage.

Possible risks: Knees, hips, low back, and shoulders.

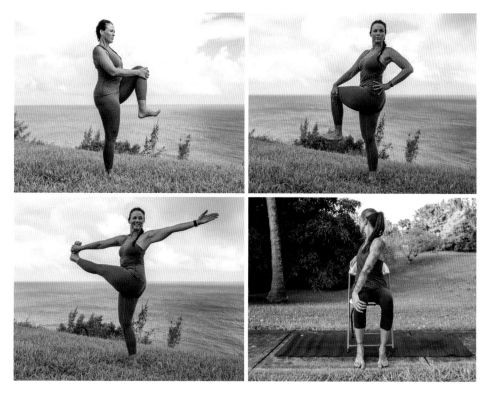

DANCER POSE

Natarajasana, known as dancer pose, is a challenging backbending standing posture. Working with the beginning variations helps strengthen the legs and back while lengthening the hip flexors, torso, and chest. Standing in mountain pose, ground into your left foot and bend your right knee, lifting the foot back toward the glutes using your hamstrings. Reach down with your right hand, taking the foot or ankle from the outside. Begin by drawing the foot close to the hip and lengthening the torso, reaching your left hand to the sky. This may be where you stay for five to eight breaths before repeating on the other side. The next stage, when you are ready, is to kick the right foot back into the hand, tip forward slightly at the hips, and reach the left arm forward. Keep the hips squared and gaze steady as you breathe. For the purposes of this book and to maintain accessibility, these are the two versions we will focus on.

Tips: To bring balance to the pose and body, focus on lifting the back leg that is in extension. Aim to square your hips and shoulders forward to reduce the twisting in the spine and open the front of the chest more.

Possible risks: Knees, low back, and shoulders.

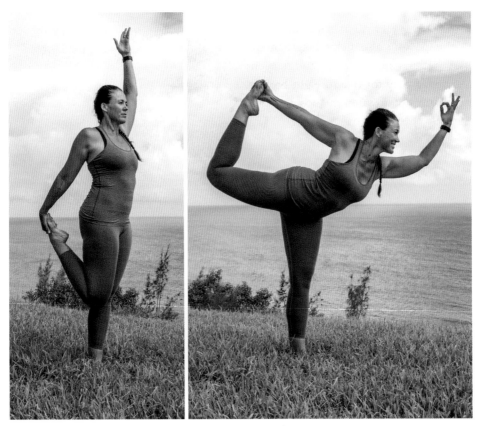

HORSE STANCE

This posture, *utkatakonasana*, known as goddess pose or horse stance, is used as a foundational stance in martial arts and is excellent for increasing external rotation of the thigh bones, building thigh and gluteal strength while lengthening the adductors of the inner thighs. From mountain pose, step your feet wide apart, facing the long edge of your mat. Turn your toes out and heels inward. Taking an inhalation to lift the core and lengthen the torso, bend your knees toward 90 degrees, pressing them wide apart. Aim to keep your torso upright, lengthening your back and drawing the front ribs inward. The hands can be at the heart in prayer pose or extended up toward the sky. Twisting from side to side in this posture also helps lengthen the back muscles and the sides, and deepens the stance. Stay for five to eight breaths, or rise up and down in the posture eight to twelve times with your breath.

Tips: Try this pose with your back against a wall to help you find an upright position. Start with your feet wide and turned out slightly with your hips, ribs, and shoulders against the wall and the legs straight. Begin to descend into the pose, pressing your hips and shoulders into the wall while bringing your ribs inward. Press your knees wide and back. When this feels comfortable, try it away from the wall.

Possible risks: Knees, low back, and shoulders.

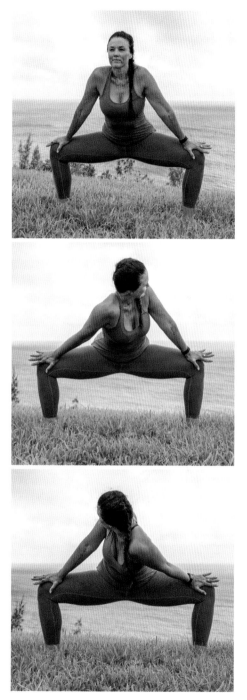

SKANDASANA

Another grounding and strengthening standing posture, *skandasana* (side lunge pose) creates mobility in the ankles and hips and extends the inner thighs and spine while challenging balance. Beginning in horse stance with the feet turned out and the knees bent deeply, push through your right foot, straightening the leg as you lower as deep as you can into the left knee and ankle in a squat. Aim to keep both feet grounded to improve ankle flexibility, and keep the torso upright with hands at the heart in prayer pose. Stay for five to eight breaths, then move to the other side.

Tips: Move side to side with the breath to get deeper into the posture. This really works ankle mobility, so take your time to get deep into it.

Possible risks: Low back, groins, and knees.

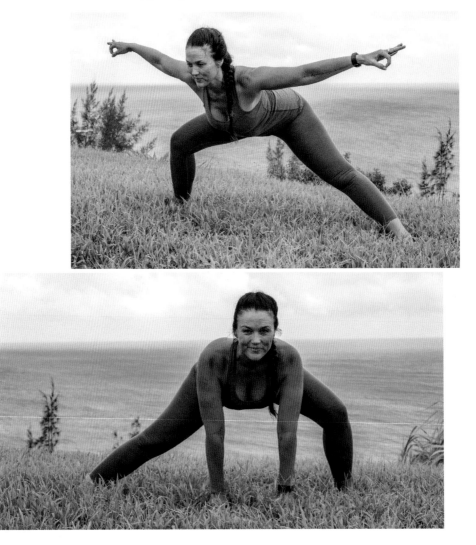

CORE POSTURES

Before we dive into core-focused postures, remember that we are defining the core as the entire torso from the floor of the pelvis to the shoulders, the sides of the body, and the low back to the top of the shoulders in back. In addition, with proper *ujayii* breathing and alignment, the deep abdominal and spinal muscles are engaged throughout the practice of yoga. On to the core-focused postures.

HOVERING TABLE

While this is not a traditional posture, it is a functional practice that is very helpful in turning on the deep core muscles at the beginning of your practice. It can be done instead of plank pose or as a preparation for plank. Starting in table posture with the hands rooting down and arms straight, tuck your toes under, lift your belly back toward your spine, spread your shoulders wide, and lift your knees about 1 to 2 inches off the ground. Hold this position while breathing. Lengthen the back of the neck and look between your hands. Keep a slight posterior tilt to your pelvis and spread the shoulders, hollowing the chest while lengthening the sternum forward. Stay for as long as you can before coming down. Work up to holding for 30 to 60 seconds.

Tips: Practice this posture at the beginning of your movement practice to turn on the core muscles of the abdominals, quadriceps, and pectorals. This builds the foundation for plank pose and four limbed staff pose.

Possible risks: Low back.

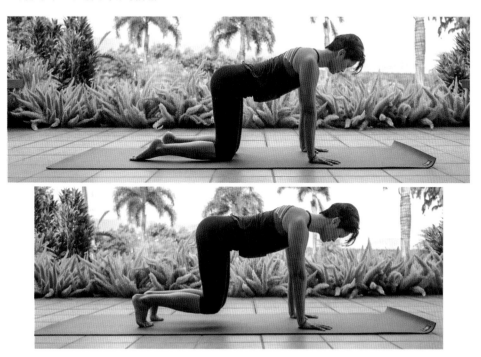

SIDE PLANK POSE

Similar to plank pose, this version engages the entire body while stabilizing length. *Vasisthasana*, side plank pose, deeply engages the sides of the hips and internal and external obliques. This pose strengthens the muscles around the shoulders while opening the chest. Beginning in plank pose, shift your weight into your right hand and lift your left hand to your left hip as you stack your hips and feet, bringing big toes together. Press down firmly into your right hand, extending from your shoulder and reaching through your hips to your feet. Lift your right hip away from the ground and extend your left arm to the sky, keeping your neck long. Gaze up toward your left hand and take five to eight breaths before switching to the second side.

Tips: Perform this posture on the forearm to take stress off the wrist if needed. The top foot can step in front of the hips as an additional grounding point.

Possible risks: Low back, shoulders, and neck.

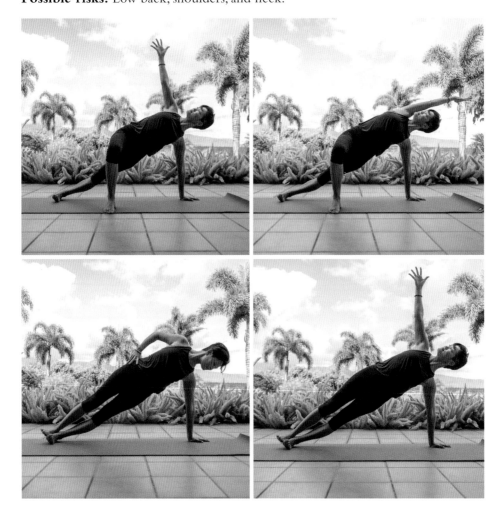

BOAT POSE

Navasana, boat pose, challenges the spinal alignment and abdominal muscles as well as the thighs. It is easy to round the spine, dropping the chest in this pose, or over-engage the hip flexors instead of balancing the engagement of the abdominals. Begin seated on the center of your sit bones with your spine long and knees bent and together, toes on the ground. Lean back a little with your hands under your hamstrings. Lift your feet, extending toes forward with shins parallel to the earth. If you can maintain the lift and length of your spine, try extending your arms forward on either side of the legs. Stay for five to ten breaths.

Tips: Work with the bent knee version for as long as you need to for strength and stability. Once this becomes easier, try extending your legs straight while lifting up through the belly and chest. Extend your hands forward alongside the legs and gaze upward toward your toes.

Possible risks: Low back and neck.

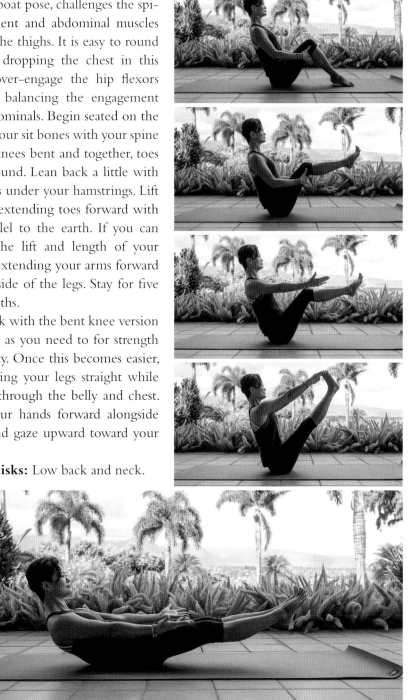

LEG LIFTS

While not a traditional pose, this is another really helpful practice that prepares the body for lifting into inversions such as shoulderstand, headstand, and plow pose. Begin by lying on your back with your arms down at your sides, pressing palms and shoulders firmly to the ground, head down. Keeping your legs extended and engaged, spine neutral, lift your right leg toward vertical on an exhalation. Inhale and bring the leg down. Repeat on the left side, alternating eight to twelve times on each side.

Tips: If this is challenging for you or causes back and neck strain, bend your knees with your toes touching the ground. Lift one knee at a time toward the sky, alternating sides.

Possible risks: Low back and neck.

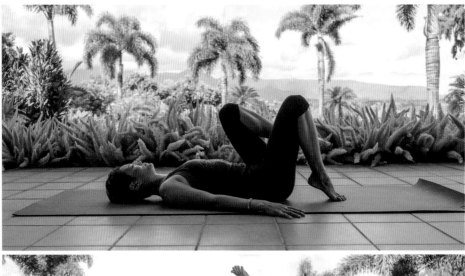

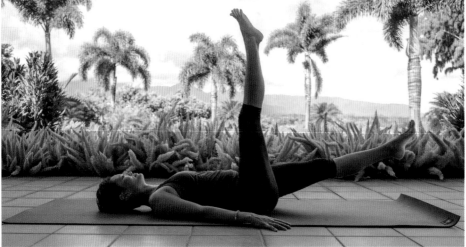

BICYCLES

Another practice that engages the abdominal muscles and hip flexors are bicycles. This targets the internal and external obliques and upper abdominals and creates a gentle twist to the spine. Begin on your back with your hands interlaced behind your head, elbows wide and knees bent. Bring your thighs perpendicular to the ground and shins parallel. On an exhalation lift your right shoulder up, reaching your elbow toward your left knee and extending your right leg out at about a 45-degree angle. Inhale as you release to center. Repeat on the other side. Alternate sides for fifteen to twenty rounds each.

Tips: One way to make the most of this pose is to reach your elbow as far past the opposite knee as possible and pause there at the end range of motion. If lifting the legs is challenging for your low back and causes pain, keep the feet on the floor with your knees bent.

Possible risks: Low back.

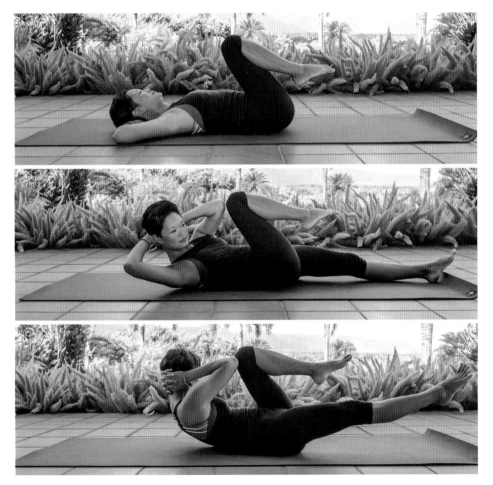

CROW POSE

Crow pose, *bakasana*, is a foundational hand balancing posture that lengthens the back of the body, stabilizes the shoulders, and engages the chest, abdominals, and thighs. Beginning in standing forward fold, squat down to place your hands flat on the ground shoulder width apart, arms inside the legs. Bend the elbows straight back, bringing upper arms toward parallel to the ground. Round your spine like cat pose while lengthening the sternum forward. Lift your knees up into your triceps as high as you can, lean forward, and keep your head up looking slightly ahead of your hands. Lift one foot at a time off the ground, squeezing your knees up and into your triceps. Extend your arms from your shoulders and breathe deeply, lifting the legs and belly up. Stay as long as you can and then rest in child's pose.

Tips: A variation of this posture that some people find easier is to have the knees on the outsides of the arms rather than in the back of the triceps. Squeeze the legs into the arms and press the arms into the legs when practicing this version.

Possible risks: Low back, shoulders, and wrists.

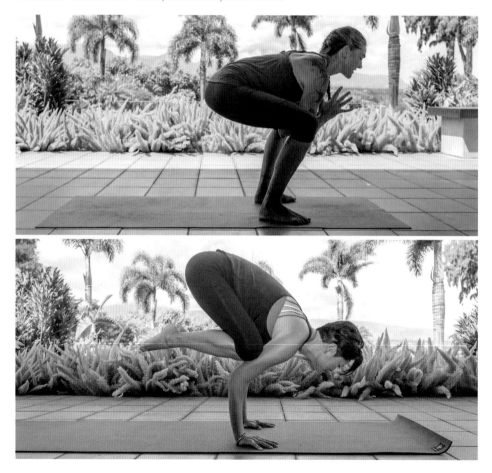

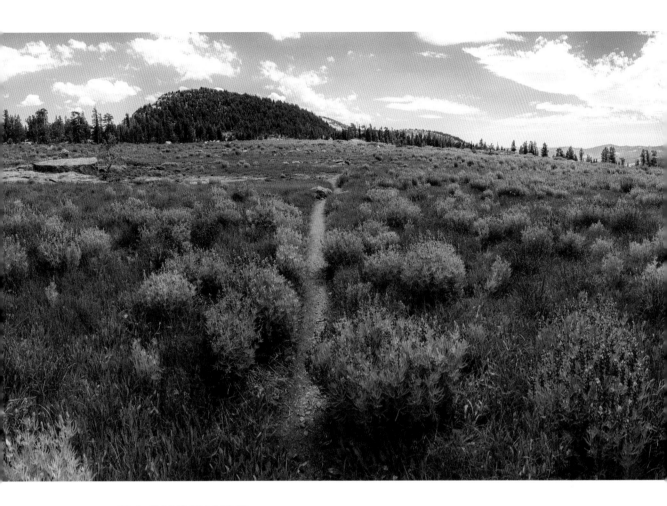

BACKBENDS

Spinal extension postures (backbends) help support the mobility, flexibility, and integrity of the spine. They lengthen the hip flexors, abdominal muscles, and chest and create more flexibility in the rib cage for easier, bigger breaths. It is important to balance the work of the upper and lower body while backbending by keeping the legs actively engaged and grounding. The gluteal muscles are extensors of the legs, so they engage during backbends. Because the gluteus maximus (the strongest muscle in the body) tends to externally rotate the thigh bones while helping with extension, it is important to hug the legs inward and aim the inner groins back while performing backbends. This creates the space to lengthen the tailbone and engage the abdominals to support the low back as well. The shoulders should draw back and down, deeply engaging the lower tips of the shoulder blades toward the spine for stability. Lastly, keep the neck long and the center of the throat moving back as you practice these postures.

LOCUST POSE

This foundational backbend, *shalabhasana*, locust pose, lengthens the spine, strengthens the muscles of the back of the body, and helps expand the chest. It is so effective for counteracting long hours of sitting and improves overall posture. Begin by lying on your belly with your arms down at your sides, palms facing upward, and legs together. On an inhalation, engage the legs, draw the shoulder blades toward each other, and extend the length of your spine through the crown of your head. As you exhale, lift your legs and engage the muscles along the back to lift your chest higher off the ground. Extend through your legs and arms as you stay in the posture, gazing slightly forward, for five to eight breaths.

Tips: Engage the shoulders back and down and press back through the head to lift the upper body. Arms can reach straight back or hands can interlace at the low back. To increase shoulder strength, extend the arms forward with the palms facing each other.

Possible risks: Low back, shoulders, and neck.

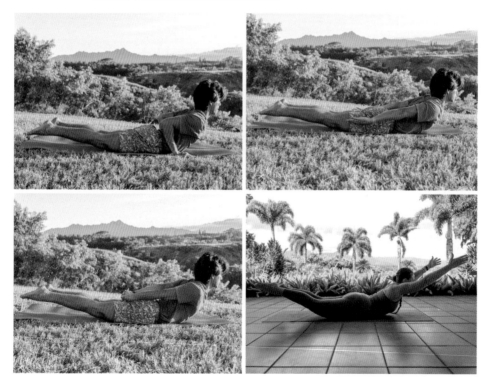

HALF FROG POSE

Ardha bekhasana, half frog posture, is an even deeper backbend that stretches the thigh muscles, abdominals, and chest, opening the front line of the body. Lie down on your belly with your elbows propped on the ground under your shoulders, forearms pressing downward, fingers spread wide. Begin lengthening your belly and chest forward and pressing your pelvis down as you bend your right knee, bringing your right foot straight up and toward the right hip. Reach back with your right hand to take the foot from the inside. Directing your right elbow toward the sky, draw the foot toward your hip to lengthen the front thigh muscles. Take five to eight breaths before repeating on the second side.

Tips: The key here is to keep your legs actively reaching back and down, both of your front hip points (ASIS) on the ground, and pressing down through your grounded arm as you reach your chest forward. Once you become comfortable with this version, you can try doing both legs at once.

Possible risks: Knees, low back, shoulders, wrists, and neck.

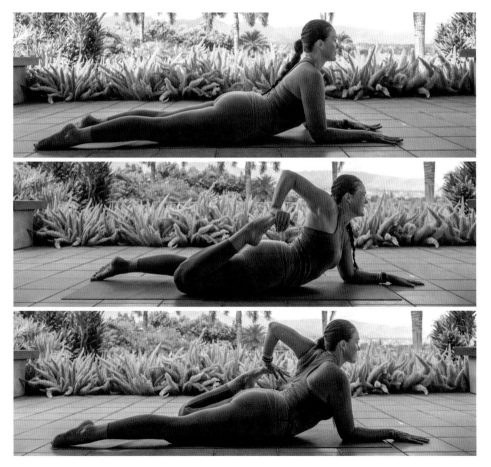

BOW POSE

This posture is said to improve digestion and lengthens the entire front of the body as you press the belly down into the earth and lift the arms and legs upward. *Dhanurasana*, bow pose, begins by lying on your belly. Bend both knees and reach back to grasp the ankles with both hands. Hug the legs toward the midline, draw your shoulders toward the spine, and on an inhalation lengthen the belly and chest forward. On an exhalation lift your thigh bones off the ground as you kick your ankles back into your hands, stretching your arms straight and gazing forward. Reach your legs up and back as you lengthen for five to eight breaths. Release back to the ground when complete.

Tips: A variation of this pose is to take hold of the outer ankles instead of the feet and press the ankles back so the thighs are flat on the ground and the shins are perpendicular to the ground. This lifts the chest up and creates a deeper backbend.

Possible risks: Knees, low back, shoulders, and neck.

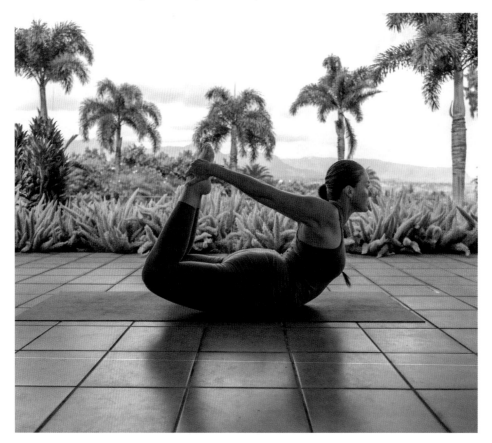

BRIDGE POSE

Setu bandha sarvangasana, bridge pose, is a very similar shape to bow pose but with a different relationship to gravity, making it a challenging backbend for many. It strengthens the hamstrings and glutes as well as the muscles along the spine and shoulders. It counteracts sitting, hiking, and kayaking wonderfully. Begin by lying on your back with your knees bent and feet hip distance apart and grounding into the floor. Extend your arms down at your sides, pressing your palms flat. Draw your shoulders close to the spine, rooting them into the ground. Inhaling, lengthen the belly and chest toward your head. On an exhalation press your feet down firmly and lift your hips up toward the sky, keeping your knees from splaying out. Press firmly into the inner edges of your feet, hugging your knees toward the midline, and press your arms and shoulders down firmly as you take five to eight breaths in the posture. Release down to active recovery pose when complete.

Tips: Try practicing this pose with a block between the upper inner thighs to help keep the inner thighs engaged and make space in the low back. Be sure to press the tops of the shoulder blades down into the earth to open the top of the chest.

Possible risks: Knees, low back, shoulders, and neck.

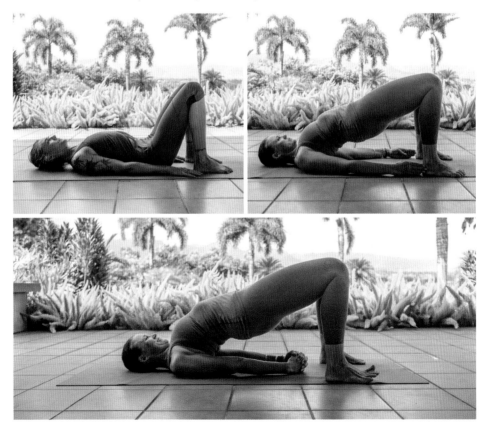

CAMEL POSE

Camel pose, *ustrasana*, is the same shape as bridge and bow pose but in an upright position. Because the shins root down and the pelvis is not fixed against the ground, the hip flexors, abdominals, and chest muscles can open more. This requires greater leg and back strength to balance the posture. Begin by kneeling with your toes tucked under. Come to standing on your knees with your thigh bones perpendicular to the ground and your shins and feet rooting down. Bring your hands to your hips, then lengthen your belly and chest upward as you roll your shoulders up and back, squeezing your elbows toward each other. On an exhalation curl your shoulders deeper onto your back as you begin to press your pelvis forward. Lift up out of your low back and lengthen your abdominal muscles with every inhalation. Draw the front ribs in and down on your exhalations. Continue to curl your shoulders and head back and press the hips forward as you reach your hands down to either the back of your thighs or your heels. It is important to keep the shins and feet rooting and the sternum lifting upward as you work in the posture. Stay for five breaths or so, continuing to extend through the neck and crown of your head and soften your gaze inward. To come out of the pose, lift the chest first and head last. Release into child's pose when complete.

Tips: It is common to drop the head back, so keep the back of the neck long and gaze forward as long as possible. You can also try this pose facing a wall with your thigh bones and hips pressing into the wall. Place your hands at chest height on the wall and press firmly to keep the chest lifting as you move up and back into the pose.

Possible risks: Knees, low back, shoulders, and neck.

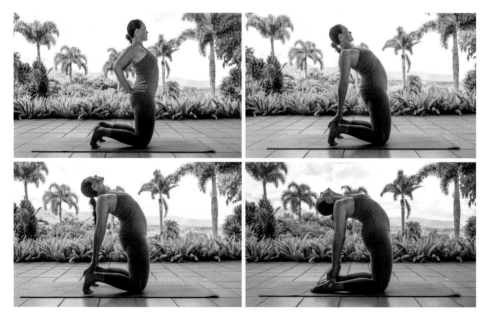

RECLINED HERO POSE

This posture is highly recommended to relieve back pain and counteract long periods of sitting. *Supta virasana*, reclined hero pose, can be a very grounding posture even though it is classified as a backbend. It targets the thigh muscles, hip flexors, and abdominal muscles. Begin in a kneeling pose, sitting on your shins with your torso upright. Lift your hips off your heels, taking your feet wider than your hips and moving the calf muscles out to the sides a bit. Sit back down with your sit bones between the heels unless this causes any knee pain or too much strain on your quadriceps muscles. If that is the case, sit on a block, a rolled hoodie or jacket, or a folded blanket just high enough to sit comfortably. Take a few breaths to settle into the pose. Once you are ready, start to walk your hands back, lengthening your abdominal muscles and chest as you ease your back down to the floor, and reaching down through your sit bones and knees to minimize arch in the lower spine. If your hips are seated on the ground, extend your arms overhead alongside your ears as you take five to eight deep breaths, lengthening. However, if you are seated up on a block

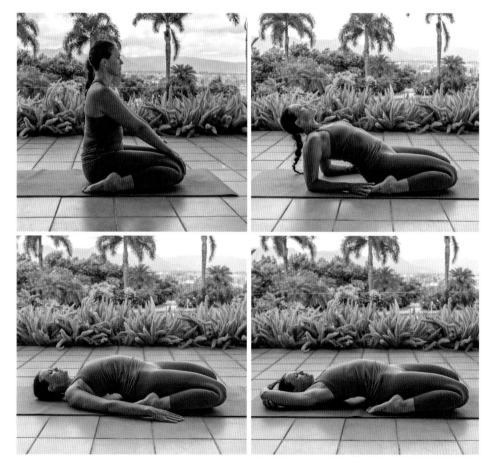

or blanket, it is best to only lower down to your elbows as far as you can and extend through the legs and chest. You may also place a folded blanket or bolster under the spine to support you in this posture.

Tips: As you begin to work with this posture, it can be helpful to work one side at a time. Extend both legs forward in seated staff pose and then fold the right leg so the heel is outside the right hip and the shin is on the ground with the knee extending forward. Release back, breathe, and lengthen the tailbone. Repeat on the other side. Then try both legs at the same time.

One nontraditional variation, toe stretching pose, involves kneeling with the toes curled under. To practice this pose, set knees under hips with shins parallel on the ground, tuck the toes under, maintaining a neutral spine and pelvis, and sit down on the heels.

Possible risks: Ankles, knees, low back, shoulders, and neck.

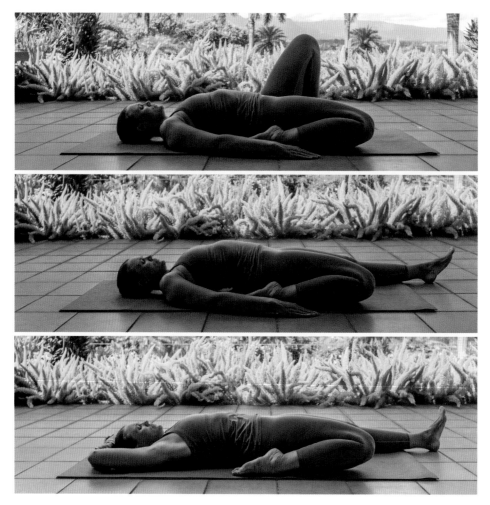

ROYAL PIGEON POSE

Royal pigeon pose, *eka pada rajakapotasana*, is both a hip opening posture and a backbend. There are multiple variations to try, but the foundation version is good for all types of athletes. It lengthens the hip flexors and iliopsoas on the back leg, the outer rotating muscles of the front hip, and the front spine while engaging the back body. Begin in downward facing dog pose then lift your right leg up. Bend the knee and bring the knee forward to just behind the right wrist with the knee bent at a 45-degree angle. The entire shin will be on the mat, with the right foot somewhere between the left wrist and the left hip. Extend the left leg back, pressing it down into the earth. Walk your hands back toward your hips while lifting the low belly, chest, and head. Root both legs downward and press the hips toward the earth as you root your tailbone and lengthen upward and curl back. Stay for five to eight breaths, then return to downward facing dog before repeating on the second side.

Tips: Work with this variation for as long as you need to, focusing on the grounding of the pelvis, the lift of the abdomen and chest, and the centering of your weight over the hips. Once this becomes comfortable and you can take at least one hand off the ground, begin to work with the deeper thigh stretch. Bend the left knee (when the right is forward) and take hold of the foot with your left hand, drawing it close

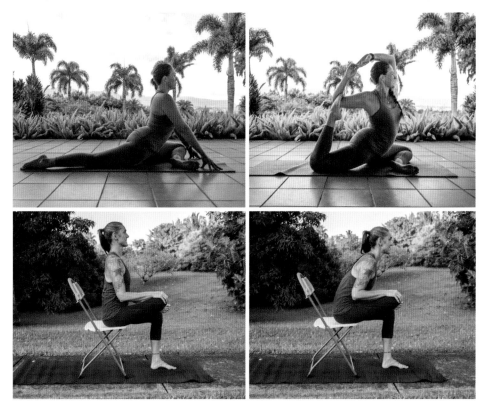

to the low back. Square your pelvis and chest forward and root down to lift upward, curling deeper.

Possible risks: Knees, low back, shoulders, and neck.

ONE-LEGGED ROYAL PIGEON POSE

Eka pada rajakapotasana, has multiple variations. Here we are focusing on the forward bending and outer hip opening version. In this posture the front leg is externally rotated with the knee bent to a 45-degree angle or so to lengthen the lateral rotators, while the back leg is fully extended with the knee down to lengthen the hip flexors. Begin in downward facing dog pose and bring the right knee forward toward your right wrist, bending the knee so that your right foot is near your left hip and your hips are rooting down toward the ground. Keeping your hips squared to the front, lengthen your front spine with an inhalation and walk your hands forward as far as is comfortable. Exhale and bow over the right shin as far as you can breathe with ease. Stay for five to eight breaths before returning to downward facing dog pose and switching sides.

Tips: If your hips don't settle down to the ground easily in this pose, you can place a blanket or block under the hip of the knee that is forward.

Possible risks: Knees, hips, and low back.

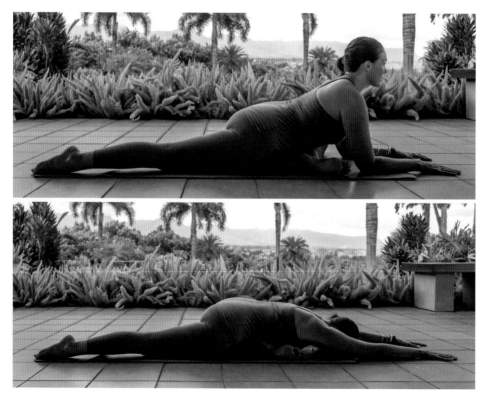

WHEEL POSE

Urdhva dhanurasana, upward facing wheel pose, is a challenging backbend that lengthens all the muscles on the front of the body and especially strengthens the shoulders and the muscles along the back, hips, and back of the legs. Begin by lying on your back with your knees bent, feet hip distance apart. Place your palms on either side of your ears with your fingers pointing toward the shoulders, hugging your elbows in slightly. Root your feet into the ground and hug inward through the adductors. Take a deep breath in, lengthening your abdominals and moving the top of your sternum toward your chin. On an exhalation press down and lift your pelvis off the ground into bridge pose, then lift your shoulders and head off the ground, pushing your arms toward straight. Stay in the posture, pressing firmly into the inner edges of your feet, lifting your pelvis, and moving your chest toward your hands to curl the upper back deeper. Let your neck lengthen and relax your jaw as you stay for five breaths or so. Release down to your back when you feel complete and extend your legs, taking a few breaths to rest.

Tips: It is often helpful to do a few repetitions of this pose to activate the back muscles, increasing warmth, opening, and strength, and add depth and freedom to the pose. Repeating two or three times helps build confidence and coordination in this complex posture.

Possible risks: Knees, low back, shoulders, neck, and wrists.

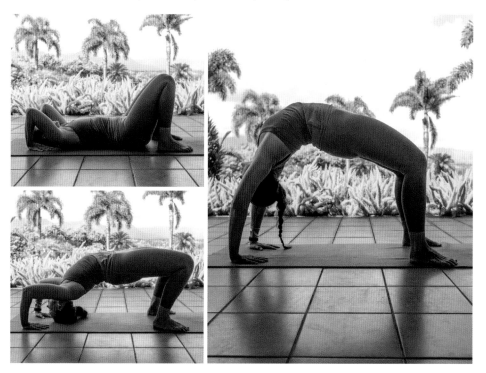

TWISTING POSTURES

Twisting postures support spinal health by lengthening both the superficial and deeper muscles that run on either side of the spine. They also help open the chest and strengthen the shoulder muscles to support an upward lift. It is important to bring the pelvis into a neutral tilt and work to minimize rounding of both the lower and upper spine. Sitting on top of a folded blanket helps create a neutral pelvis. As you revolve around your center, only go as far as you can take deep breaths. Complete the spinal twists by turning your head toward the shoulder on the side of the twist and soften your gaze downward. Twists are said to bring us into our center and help focus a wandering mind.

SIMPLE SEATED TWIST

This seated twist, *parivritta sukhasana*, is perfect to warm up the spine as well as a counterpose at the end of a backbending practice to re-center your awareness. Begin by taking a simple cross-legged seat. If your pelvis tips back and your spine rounds, sit up on a folded blanket or a block to lift the pelvis above the knees. On an inhalation lift the spine and the left arm toward the sky. As you exhale, place your right hand behind your right hip and your left hand on your right knee, twisting the torso to the right. As you inhale, continue to lift upward and send your breath into the back of your lungs, turning your gaze past your right shoulder. Stay for five to eight breaths before returning to center and repeating on the second side.

Tips: Initiate the twist from deep in your belly, slowly revolving around the spine as you engage your core. Continue lengthening up the spine, twisting through the shoulders and lastly the neck.

Possible risks: Knees, low back, and neck.

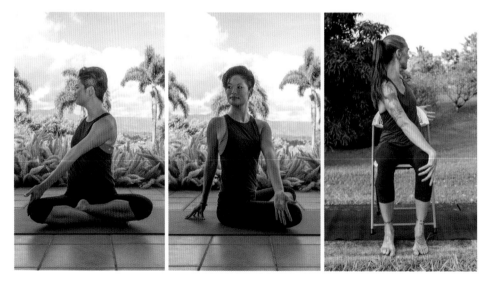

MARICHYASANA

Named after the yogic sage Marichi, this deep spinal twist lengthens the outer hip muscles and opens the chest. There are a few different variations of this posture possible—we will cover the most accessible one, *Marichyasana C*. From a seated posture extend the left leg out in front of you and bend the right knee, placing the foot on the ground near the right sit bone. Inhaling, lengthen the front spine and left side body as you extend your left arm overhead. On an exhalation cross the left elbow outside the right knee and place the right hand on the ground near the right hip. Rotate your torso toward the right as you breathe, expanding the back and lifting upward through the spine. Gaze past the right shoulder as you take five to eight breaths. Return to center and switch legs to repeat on the left side.

Tips: As with the previous twist, you may try taking the arm around the bent knee as opposed to the outside of the knee for an easier and more spacious pose. It is also helpful to practice this pose seated next to a wall, with the hip of the bent knee close to the wall. Place your hands on the wall to leverage the twist.

Possible risks: Knee, low back, and neck.

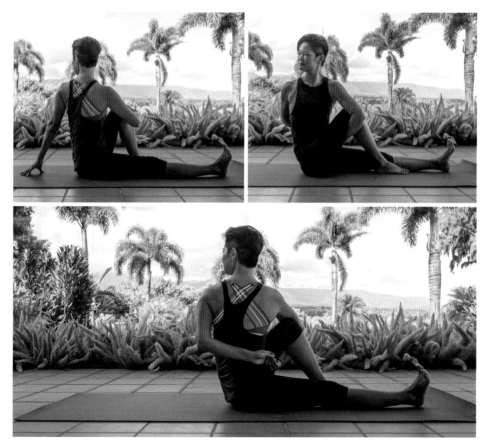

HALF LORD OF THE FISH POSE

Ardha matseyandrasana is a deeper twist that deepens the internal rotation of the leg you are twisting toward, lengthens the outer hip and spinal muscles, and opens the chest. Beginning in an easy sitting posture, bend your right knee, bringing your foot in close to your right sit bone. Cross your left foot toward your right outer hip. Inhaling, lift your left arm up, getting as long as you can in the side and front of the body. Twist the torso to the right, placing your left elbow on the outside of your right knee and pressing your right hand on the ground behind you. Look past your right shoulder, lengthening your spine as you take five to eight breaths here. Release to center, switch legs, and repeat on the second side.

Tips: An easier and more accessible version of this pose has the left arm (when the right knee is bent toward the sky) wrap around the knee instead of crossing to the outside of the knee. Hug the knee inward as you twist toward the right and press your back hand (right one) into the ground to keep the spine long.

Possible risks: Knees, low back, shoulders, and neck.

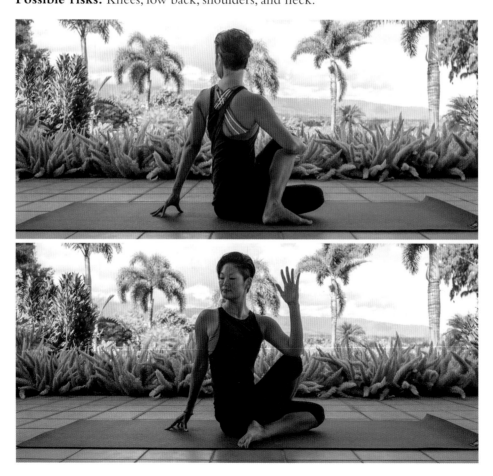

BHARADVAJASANA

Named after the Hindu teacher Bharadvaja, this twist looks deceptively easy and combines outer hip opening with deep spinal twisting. Begin in a kneeling posture with your toes untucked. Shift your hips over to the right to sit on the floor or a prop next to your feet. Ground your pelvis evenly or sit on a folded blanket to level the hips. Sit up tall, pressing your right hand outside the left knee, palm facing upward if possible. Inhaling, lengthen the spine upward and wrap your left arm around behind your back, catching the outer right hip. As you exhale, turn your head and gaze back toward the right shoulder. Stay for five to eight breaths before releasing to center and repeating on the second side.

Tips: If your sit bones are not evenly weighted or you feel you are tipping far to one side unable to center the spine, sit up on the edge of a blanket or block.

Possible risks: Knees, low back, and neck.

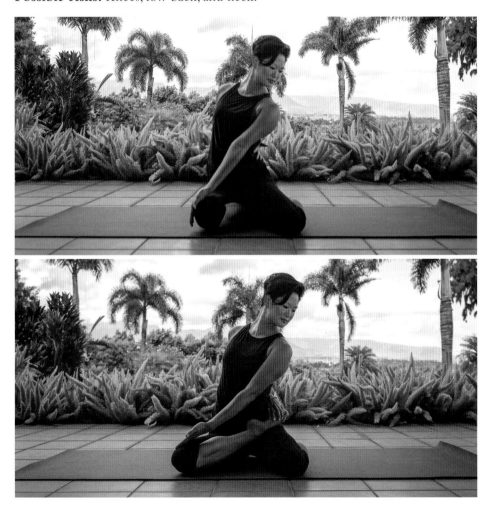

JATTHARA PARVATTASANA

Supine twists are a wonderful way to wind down at the end of practice. This posture is fairly accessible and helpful at relieving low back pain while it gently lengthens the spine and opens the chest, as the name *jatthara* (abdomen) *parva* (turning) suggests. Begin by lying on your back with your knees bent, feet on the floor. On an inhalation draw your knees to your chest and take your arms out wide in a "T" position. Extend your legs fully, squeezing them toward the midline and extending through the toes. Inhale and press your hands and shoulders downward, then exhale to take your legs over to the left toward the ground. Continue to press down through your arms and pelvis, extending through your legs, as you take five to eight breaths. Inhale to return to center and repeat toward the right.

Tips: As you begin to practice this posture or if you have low back pain, bend your knees to a 90-degree angle or so. Focus on expanding across the chest by pressing both shoulders down. If your knees do not touch the floor with both shoulders down, place a bolster or blanket under the knees for support.

Possible risks: Low back, shoulders, and neck.

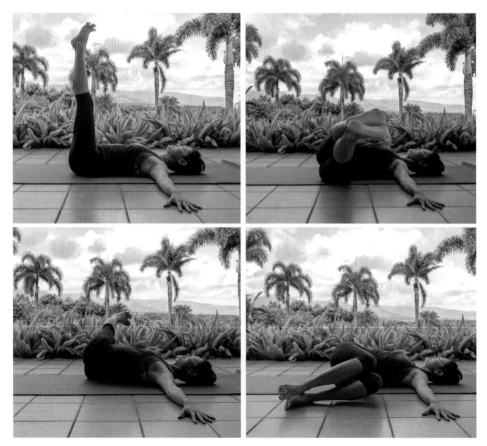

SIDE-BENDING POSTURES

Postures that lengthen the lateral sides of the body from the hips through the shoulders are extremely beneficial for all outdoor athletes. These postures help lengthen the psoas, abdominals, chest, and shoulders as well as the quadratus lumborum muscles on the low back and the muscles along the spine. The side we are bending to shortens, contracting the muscles of the side waist and the stabilizers of the shoulders. Climbers and paddlers use these movements in their sport while hikers, backpackers, snowboarders, skiers, and cyclists will find these postures excellent for rounding out and balancing their bodies. The low back, shoulders, and neck are potential risk areas for side-bending postures. Proceed carefully if you are sensitive in any of those areas.

EASY SIDE-BENDING POSE

If you are beginning your practice seated or are in a chair, canoe, kayak, or on a bike for long periods, this is a great pose. It has similar benefits to standing crescent pose (described above), with the addition of a little more hip opening as you are seated. Begin in easy sitting pose, *sukhasana*. Inhale the arms overhead and lengthen the torso upward, then on an exhalation take the left hand down to the ground out at your left side. Reach your right arm overhead, extending the right side body. Look past your right arm to open the chest as you take five breaths. Return to center on an inhalation then repeat, extending toward the right side. Keep your hips rooting down as you perform this posture, your neck long, and your face relaxed.

Tips: If your low back rounds in easy sitting pose, then sit on a folded blanket so that your knees are below your hips. This will help lift and align the spine.

Possible risks: Sacroiliac dysfunction, shoulders, and neck.

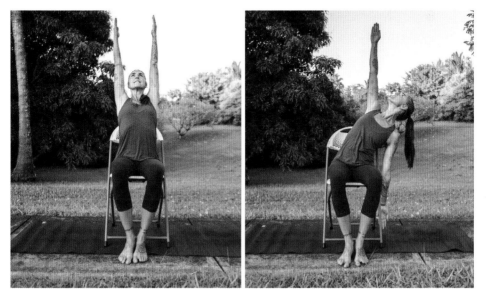

SIDE-BENDING CHILD'S POSE

Prasarita balasana, side-bending child's pose, is another accessible and effective side-bending posture. This one increases the forward bending and lengthening of the back muscles and outer hips. Begin in child's pose with your knees wide apart and your arms extending on the ground in front of you. On an inhalation lift the torso slightly, walk your hands over toward the left on the ground as far as you can, and place your forehead on the mat or a block. As you exhale, lengthen the back over your left thigh, reaching your sternum toward the knee and keeping your right hip on the ground. Stay for five breaths, then return through center on an inhalation. Repeat toward the right thigh, staying for five breaths once you get into the posture.

Tips: If bending your knees deeply and sitting back is difficult, place a folded blanket between your hamstrings and calves or sit up on a block.

Possible risks: Low back, sacroiliac dysfunction, knees, shoulders, and neck.

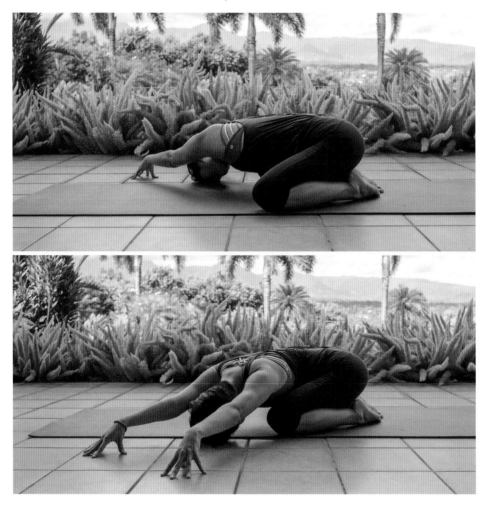

GATE POSE

Parighasana, gate pose, is a deeper side stretch that lengthens the front of the body, sides, and back as well as the adductors (inner thigh muscles) on the extended leg, preparing you for standing postures. Begin by kneeling with your toes untucked. Come up to the knees and extend your left leg out to the side, placing the left foot on the ground with the outer edge parallel to the mat. Ground through the right knee, shin, and top of the foot while you simultaneously extend out of the left hip through the left foot. Inhale and take your arms out to your sides, lengthening your torso. As you exhale, bend the torso to the left, take your left hand down the left thigh as far as it will go, and extend your right arm alongside your face. Turn your gaze toward the right arm to open the chest and shoulder muscles and lengthen the upper spine. Stay for five breaths, then return to center, switch legs, and repeat, extending toward the right leg.

Tips: Keep your hips level with the earth in this pose, and use your breath to lengthen the sides of the body.

Possible risks: Low back, shoulders, and neck.

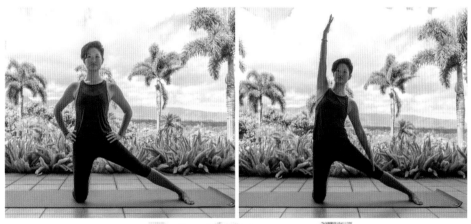

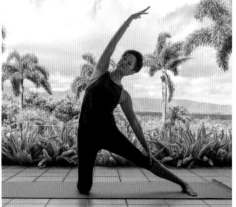

SIDE-BENDING WIDE LEGGED POSE

This seated posture, *parivritta upa vistha konasana*, lengthens the hamstrings, inner thigh muscles, sides of the body, shoulders, and back while contracting the abdominal muscles, thighs, and stabilizers of the shoulder you are bending toward. This is one of the few postures that lengthens the deep iliopsoas muscles along with the quadratus lumborum. Begin by sitting on the ground with your legs open wide as far as you can take them. Turn the legs in so the toes are pointing upward and the heels are rooting down. Bring the pelvis to a neutral position so you are sitting on the center of your sit bones or, if needed, use a folded blanket under the hips to allow the pelvis and spine to lift upward without rounding. Keeping the legs rooting and actively lifting through your torso, extend your arms out to the sides. On an exhalation, bend left and reach your left arm toward your left leg, holding either the ankle or foot. Extend the right arm alongside your face, keeping the hips rooted. Take five to eight breaths as you gaze under the right arm. Inhale to release to center and exhale to extend toward your right foot to repeat on the second side.

Tips: For a variation of this posture that extends the side as well as the back even more, try twisting toward one leg and bending forward toward the knee. As with all twists and forward bends, keep the sit bones rooting and draw the low belly up and in.

Possible risks: Low back, sacroiliac dysfunction, shoulders, and neck.

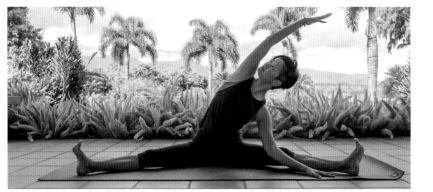

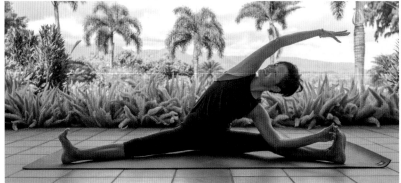

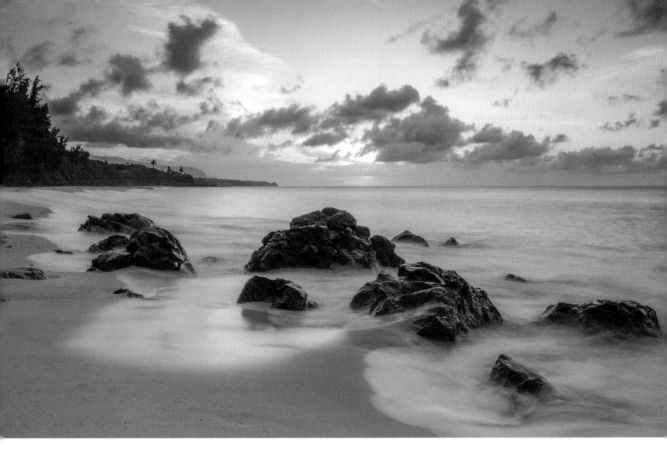

HIP OPENING POSTURES

Since the pelvis has so many different muscles with different functions that attach to it, this class of postures is fairly large and complex. Keep in mind that in some ways all yoga postures help to balance the hips, both stabilizing and opening different groups of muscles. All standing postures prepare the body for deeper hip opening as well. As we noted in the anatomy section, knee health is related to hip health and pelvic alignment. If you have injured or sore knees, practice with caution as you work with these poses. All of our adventure sports challenge the hip muscles, and everyone benefits from bringing some hip opening postures into their practice. That being said, remember that we are all unique and our bone structures and personal histories will determine how far we go in postures. For instance, in cobbler's pose, one person may have their knees on the ground and easily be able to extend the torso forward toward the ground while another student (even within the same sport) may have their knees up away from the ground and struggle to extend forward at all. Be not only patient with yourself but also realistic. Injuries in yoga often come when we push ourselves beyond where our joints can go in an attempt to make our pose look like someone else's. This is your practice and your pelvis, and injuries take a long time to heal and take us away from the activities we love.

EASY SITTING POSE

Sukhasana, easy sitting pose, is a common posture often used for meditation. Both thigh bones are externally rotated and the inner thighs lengthen. The pelvis is neutral as you sit on the center of your sit bones, and the spine lengthens upward in its natural curves. As you extend forward, the glutes and back muscles, sides, and chest all lengthen. Begin by sitting on the ground with your legs extended forward. Bend your right knee, turning the thigh outward and crossing your right ankle in toward the left sit bone. Then bend the left knee, turning the thigh outward and crossing the ankle under the right knee. Take an inhalation to lengthen the torso upward, then walk your hands forward as far as you can, bending forward. Stay with your neck long and face relaxed for five to eight breaths. Return to sitting, switch the cross of your legs and repeat on the second side.

Tips: If your low back rounds in this posture, sit up on a folded blanket or bolster to lift the hips so the knees can release toward the floor. Keep your feet actively engaged and root down through your sit bones.

Possible risks: Knees and low back.

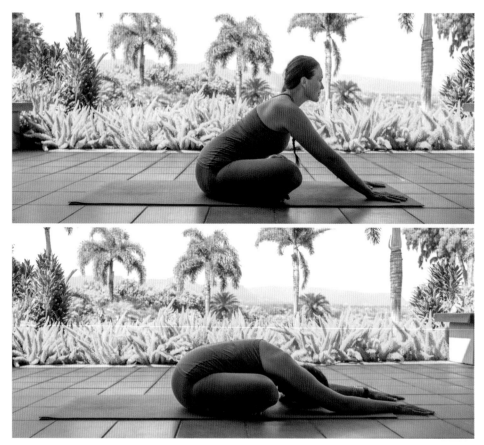

LIZARD LUNGE

While not a traditional posture, *utthan pristhasana*, lizard lunge, is a deep low lunge and both a strong forward fold and hip extension. It lengthens the inner thigh muscles and back along with the glutes and hip flexors. This posture is the foundation for many deeper hip openers, forward folds, and hand balancing postures. Begin in low lunge with the right foot forward and the left foot back with the toes tucked under. The back knee can stay grounded, or you can straighten the back leg for a deeper expression. Take your hands down to the ground on the inside of your right foot, moving the foot out to the side a few inches. Keep your legs and core actively engaged as you push back through your left heel and extend your spine forward. Stay for five to eight breaths before stepping forward to switch sides.

Tips: When you feel ready, you can lower your forearms down to a block or the ground to take this posture deeper. Keep the belly lifting up and in during this posture to support the low back and further lengthen the hip flexors.

Possible risks: Low back, groins, knees, and neck.

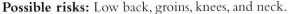

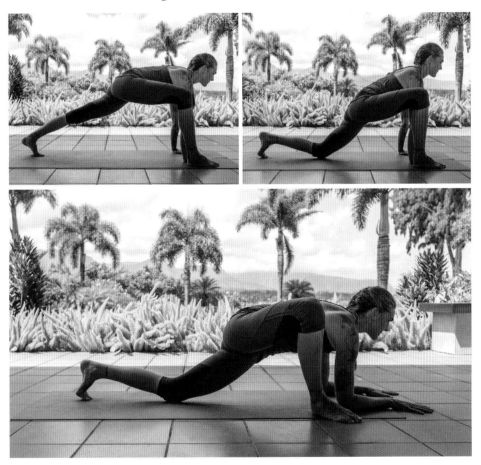

TWISTED THIGH STRETCH

Parivritta utthan pristhasana, twisted thigh stretch, is another modern posture; this one is essential for hikers, backpackers, and paddlers of all kinds. In addition to the benefits of low lunge, it lengthens the quadriceps muscles and iliopsoas while also opening the chest and strengthening the shoulders. Begin in low lunge with your right foot forward and left leg back with the knee down. Keep the low belly engaged, pressing the hips forward as you place the left hand on the inside of your right foot and the right hand on your right knee. Begin to lengthen your torso as you twist toward the right shoulder, opening the chest. Bend your left knee and reach your right hand back to take hold of the foot. Draw your belly back, lengthen through the sternum, and bring your left foot in close to your hip as you take five to eight breaths. Release to lizard lunge or to forward fold before stepping the right foot back for the second side.

Tips: If bending the knee deeply creates pain in the joint, try pressing the foot back into the hand and opening the knee joint more. This also creates a deeper opening through the chest.

Possible risks: Low back, knees, and shoulders.

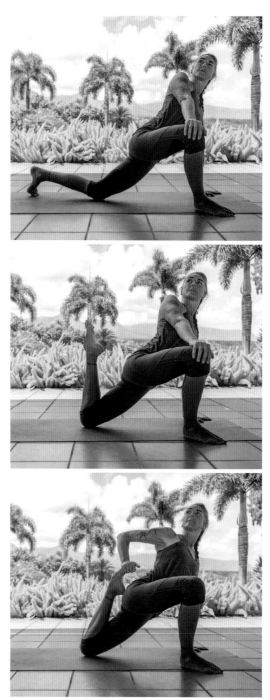

SEATED STAFF POSE

This is one of those postures that looks easy but is deceptively challenging for the back of the legs and hip muscles. *Dandasana*, seated staff pose, is the foundation for all seated postures. With the pelvis fixed on the ground and the spine upright, the hamstrings stretch as the thighs, core, and back muscles all engage. Begin by sitting on the ground with your legs extended in front of you. Bring the inseam of your legs together, rooting your heels down and stretching your toes toward the sky, hands on either side of your hips. Actively root your heels and sit bones down, finding a neutral pel-

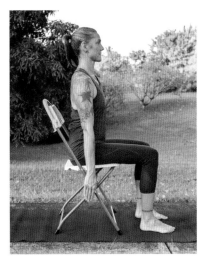

vis, while you push the hands down and elongate through the torso and crown of the head. Draw the shoulders back and down and drop your chin toward your chest. Stay for five to eight breaths before releasing.

Tips: If your pelvis tips back and your spine rounds in this posture, sit up on the edge of a folded blanket to create more mobility in the pelvis and regain neutral curves in the spine.

Possible risks: Knees, hamstrings, and low back.

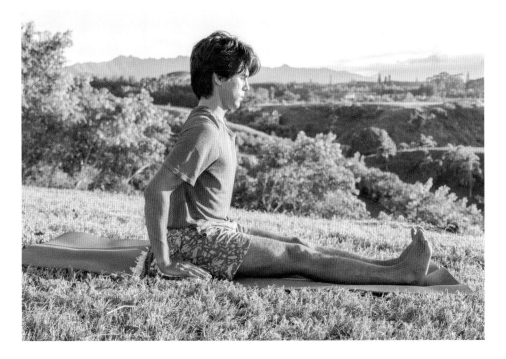

GARLAND POSE

Squatting is one of the natural human movements that many modern humans have lost the capacity for. Most children can drop down into a squat to play and rest with ease, while most adults do not even attempt it. With practice and patience, we can regain the mobility of the ankles, hips, and spine and receive the benefits of this posture. *Malasana*, garland pose, stretches the ankles, calves, thighs, and hips and lengthens the spine while engaging the core and shoulders. Begin in mountain pose with your feet slightly wider than hip distance apart. Turn the feet out slightly to create more space in the hip joint. Take a breath in, lifting up through the abdominals and chest, then squat down as far as you can while keeping your heels on the ground and your torso upright. Stay for five breaths or so, then return to mountain pose.

Tips: If your heels want to lift up when you squat down, try either placing a block under your hips to keep you lifted with the heels down or placing a folded blanket under the heels to ground into.

Possible risks: Knees and low back.

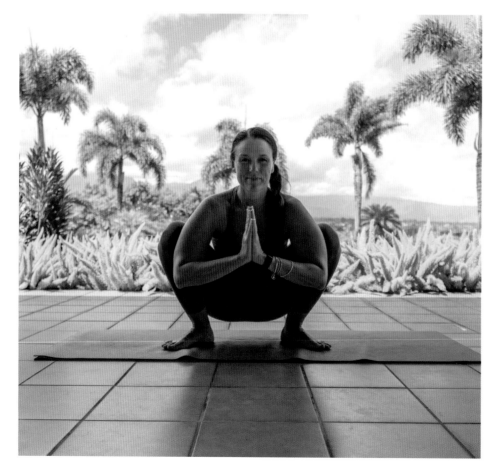

LEAPING MONKEY POSE

Hanumanasana, leaping monkey posture, is a deep hip opening pose that lengthens the hamstrings and glutes on the front leg while stretching the hip flexors and engaging the hamstrings and glutes on the back leg. Begin in a low lunge posture with the right foot forward and left leg back with the knee down. With your hands propped on the ground or blocks, begin to extend your right leg, reaching the foot forward as you reach back through the left leg. Keep squaring your pelvis forward by internally rotating your left thigh and drawing your right thigh bone back in. Lift up through the low belly and extend through your crown as you take three to five breaths. This posture takes patience and practice, don't rush into it—rather, take your time to work with it.

Tips: Your hands may stay on the ground or blocks if you are new to this pose or it is challenging. One variation of the pose extends the arms overhead along either side of the face with the gaze slightly upward.

Possible risks: Knees, hamstrings, groins, and low back.

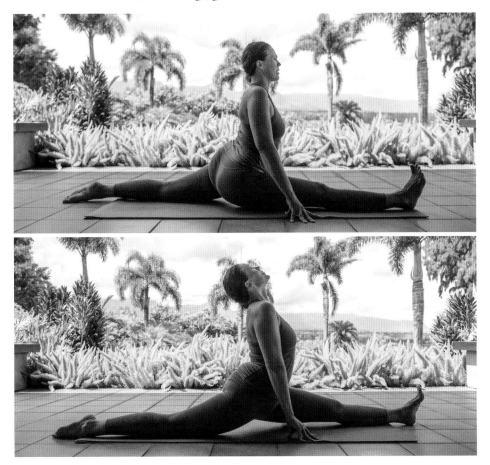

COW FACED POSE

This posture, *gomukhasana*, has two phases—the first is the deep outer hip opening and the second is the shoulder stretch. Begin by sitting in a seated staff pose. Bend your left knee, externally rotate the thigh bone, and bring your left foot to the outside of your right hip. Then bend the right knee, crossing it over the left and placing the foot to the outside of the left hip. Sit upright with your hands on the ground or walking them out in front of you, taking five to eight breaths before switching sides. This pose lengthens the outer hip muscles and iliotibial band (ITB) to allow the pelvis to ground. Once the pelvis is squarely rooted and the foundation of the posture is more comfortable, try adding the shoulder stretch, which stretches the chest and back of the shoulder on one side while lengthening the chest, triceps, and latissimus dorsi on the opposite side.

For this second phase of the posture, keep the torso upright and extend your left arm upward, bending at the elbow as you reach your left hand down in between the shoulder blades. Keeping your right arm at your side (internally rotated), bend the elbow and reach the hand up toward the shoulders blades to clasp the left fingers if possible. If clasping is challenging, use a strap, shirt, or bandana between the hands. Keep your legs actively hugging toward the midline as you ground the pelvis and lengthen through the torso, reaching the elbows in opposite directions as you breathe. Stay for five to eight breaths before switching to the opposite side.

Tips: If crossing your knees is challenging or one hip is floating above the ground as you try this posture, sit on a folded blanket or block to stay upright in the posture rather than folding forward.

Possible risks: Knees, low back, and shoulders.

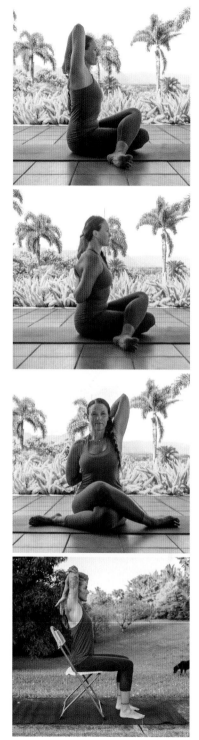

SEATED BABY CRADLE

Traditionally a preparation for a deeper posture, the basic form of this pose is accessible and has benefits for all athletes, especially hikers, cyclists, and paddlers. In *hindolasana*, seated baby cradle, the focus is on lengthening the outer rotator muscles of the hip as well as the spine. Begin in seated staff pose with the spine erect. Bend your right knee to a 90-degree angle and, using both hands, lift the shin toward your chest with the knee pointed outward and draw the right foot toward the midline, externally rotating the right hip. As much as possible, keep the spine erect and the shoulders drawing down and back slightly as you stay for five to eight breaths. Release to staff pose and continue to the other side.

Tips: If this pose is challenging for you, try rocking side to side, massaging the outer hip to help release the tension. Once you can get your shin parallel to the floor, you can slide your forearms under the shin and lift up through the spine as you hug the leg toward the chest.

Possible risks: Knees, hamstrings, and shoulders.

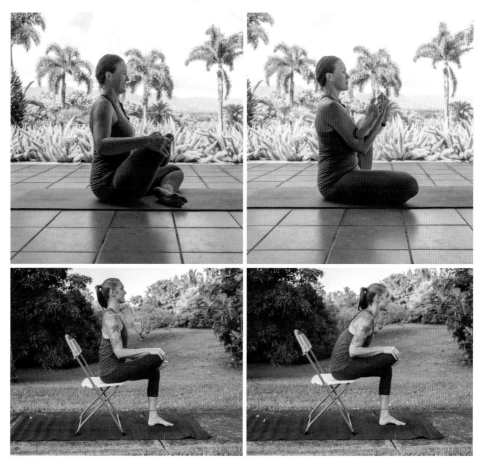

FIRE LOG POSE

Agni stambhasana, fire log pose, builds upon seated baby cradle by increasing the external rotation of both thigh bones, lengthening the gluteal muscles and the back. Begin in easy sitting pose with your pelvis neutral. Lean back on your hands and shift both heels forward until your shins are parallel with each other. Tip the pelvis forward until you can sit upright again, then fold forward as far as is comfortable with your hands in front of you. Once this is comfortable, stack the right ankle on top of the left knee and repeat the forward fold, staying for five to eight breaths. Repeat on the other side, placing the left ankle on top of the right knee and folding forward. Keep the legs and core engaged in this posture to stabilize the knees and low back.

Tips: If sitting up tall without the low back rounding is a challenge, sit on the edge of a blanket or bolster to support the spinal lift.

Possible risks: Knees, hips, and low back.

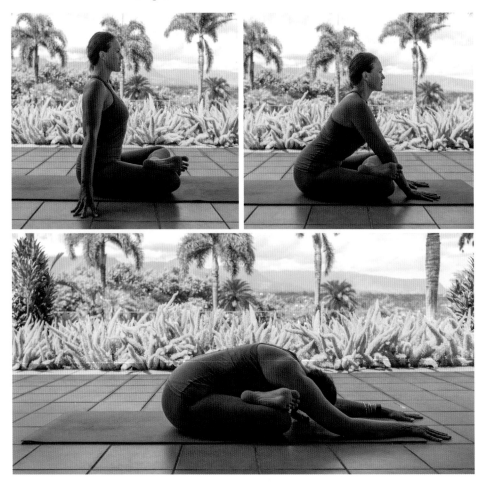

LOTUS POSE

The quintessential yoga posture, *padmasana*, is no joke, especially for cyclists, runners, hikers, and paddlers of all kinds. *Padmasana*, lotus pose, requires deep external rotation of both thigh bones; mobility in the ankles, hips, and low back; strong healthy knees; and great patience. That being said, working toward this posture creates a balanced and stable foundation for sitting in meditation and finding stillness in challenging times. The previous hip opening postures lay the groundwork for this one.

Begin by sitting in easy crossed-legged posture with the spine erect. Lift your right foot up in a point and draw the foot up into the left hip crease. Inhaling, lift up through your spine and crown, placing both hands on the knees, palms down with the arms straight. Close your eyes and take five to eight breaths before repeating on the other side. Work here in half lotus pose first, then move on to full lotus if that makes sense for your body and life. It isn't for everyone.

Once comfortable in half lotus, begin to work on full lotus. For this, draw the right foot into the left hip crease, then lean to the left and bring the left foot into the right hip crease. The hips will be externally rotated, the shins will be crossed, and both feet will be on top of the legs, soles facing upward. Rest the hands on the knees, sit upright, and close your eyes as you take five to ten breaths. Repeat on the second side with the right shin on top of the left. Classically, the right foot is always brought in first, but balance is key so make sure you work both sides.

Keep in mind that hip mobility is largely determined by the shape and size of the bones in the hip joint. Flexibility will increase with practice, but only to the degree that the bones allow for movement. Be patient and careful with this posture as the knees will take the pressure of any forcing into the pose.

Tips: If the top knee does not come down to the ground with ease once you get into the pose or if there is pain, place a thin blanket under the knee for support.

Possible risks: Ankles, knees, hips, and low back.

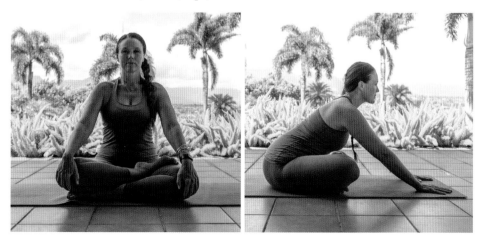

FORWARD FOLDING POSTURES

Forward bends are postures that stretch the back of the legs, glutes, and muscles along the back of the body and back of the neck. The front of the body is engaged to balance and encourage the lengthening of the back body. As with twisting postures it is important to bring the pelvis into a neutral tilt. Sitting on a folded blanket helps bring the pelvis to neutral for seated poses. It is important to lengthen the belly and sternum forward when working with these poses to balance the postures. They are known for drawing the awareness inward, calming the nervous system, and quieting the mind. The key is to remember the balance of *sthira* and *sukha*, effort and ease.

RUNNER'S STRETCH

Ardha hanumanasana, also known as runner's stretch, is a beginning forward folding posture that lengthens the hamstrings on the front leg, the glutes, and the back muscles. Begin in a low lunge with the right foot forward and the left leg back with the knee down. Move your hips back so that your left thigh bone is perpendicular to the ground and your hands are on either side of you. Extend the right leg straight, digging your heel in the ground with the foot flexed, toes to the sky. Inhale and lengthen through the front body, lifting the low belly and extending through the sternum as you bow forward over the right leg. Stay for five to eight breaths before switching to the other side.

Tips: If your back tends to round in this posture, place blocks under your hands to lift up and lengthen through the spine.

Possible risks: Hamstrings and low back.

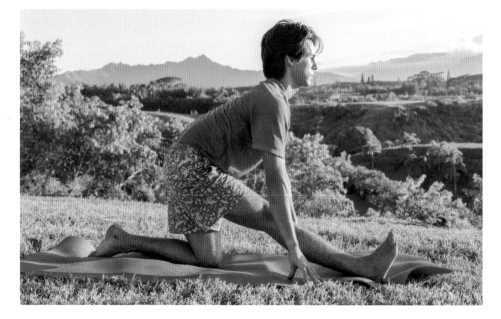

HEAD TO KNEE POSE

This seated forward fold adds a hip opening element to the hamstring and back lengthening of a forward fold. *Janu sirsasana*, head to knee pose, targets the deep quadratus lumborum muscles that lie on either side of the spine connecting from the top of the posterior pelvis to the lower ribs. Begin in seated staff pose, then bend the right knee, bringing the inside of the foot to press the inner left thigh, close to the inner groin, with the knee out to the side. Ground through the sit bones, tilting the pelvis forward, and extend fully through the left leg, rooting the heel with the foot flexed. Inhale and extend the spine, lifting the low belly as you twist toward the left knee. Reach your hands forward to the ankle, foot, or either side of the leg as you bow forward. Take five to eight breaths before returning to seated staff pose and switching sides.

Tips: If the knee does not touch the earth, prop it up with a blanket for support.

Possible risks: Hamstrings, knees, and low back.

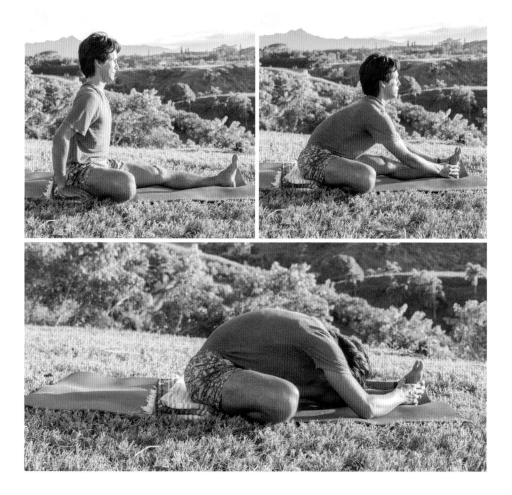

COBBLER'S POSE

Badha konasana, bound angle or cobbler's pose as it is commonly known, is a deep forward fold that includes external rotation of the thigh bones to lengthen the back of the hip muscles as well as the spine. Start in seated staff pose, then bend both knees out to the side, bringing the soles of the feet together as close to the inner groins as is comfortable. Prop your hands on the ground next to you, lengthening through the torso and pressing your feet together, rooting your outer thighs toward the earth. As you exhale, lengthen forward as much as you can, keeping the front spine long, allowing your neck to lengthen and relax. Stay for five to eight breaths before releasing.

Tips: If you have knee pain or the knees are high above the ground, prop them with blocks or blankets. Likewise, if tipping the pelvis forward and lengthening the front spine is challenging, lift the pelvis onto a folded blanket so the knees can drop.

Possible risks: Knees, hips, and low back.

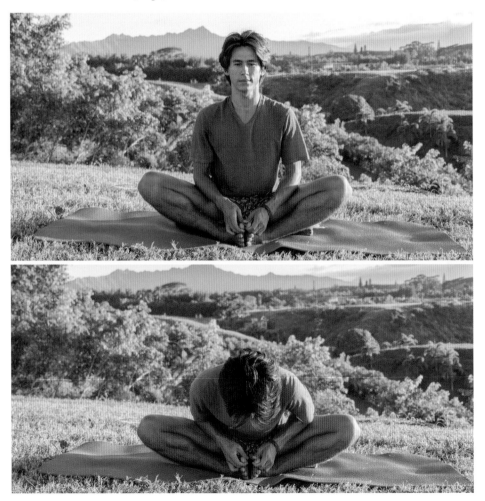

SEATED FORWARD FOLD

Moving from seated staff pose, *paschimottanasana*, seated forward fold, is a deeper forward bend that stretches the back of the legs, glutes, and the entire back through the base of the skull. Begin seated in staff pose with the legs hugging the midline and rooting down. Inhale and lengthen the spine upward, lifting the low belly and sternum, then reach forward and take hold of your ankles or feet. Keep your thighs and core engaged as you stay. Breathe deeply five to eight times before releasing out of the pose.

Tips: If your low back rounds in this posture, sit on a folded blanket and use a strap around the feet held in each hand. This will allow you to tilt the pelvis forward more and lengthen through the front of the spine.

Possible risks: Hamstrings, hips, and low back.

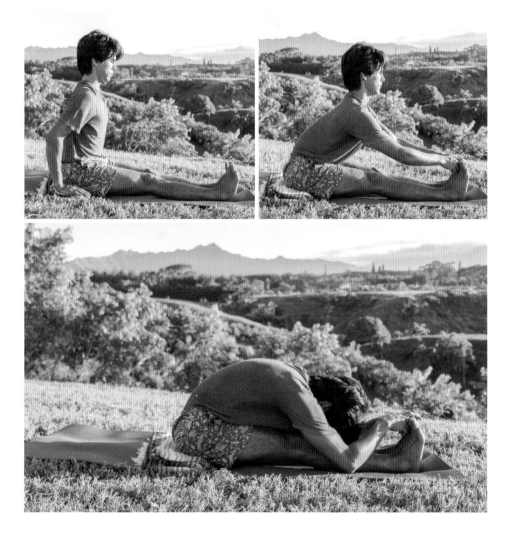

SEATED WIDE LEGGED FORWARD FOLD

Upavistha konasana, seated wide legged forward fold, is another deep posture that lengthens the inner thigh muscles as well as the back of the legs, hips, and back of the torso. Begin by sitting in staff pose, then take your feet as wide apart as you can, keeping the backs of your legs rooting and your toes pointing toward the sky. With your hands behind you, tip your pelvis forward as far as you can. Inhale and lengthen the abdominals and sternum. Bow forward on an exhalation, placing your hands out in front of you. Stay for five to ten breaths, keeping your legs, belly, and shoulders actively engaged.

Tips: If your low back rounds in this posture, sit on a folded blanket and use a strap around the feet held in each hand. This will allow you to tilt the pelvis forward more and keep the spine long as you fold forward.

Possible risks: Hamstrings, hips, and low back.

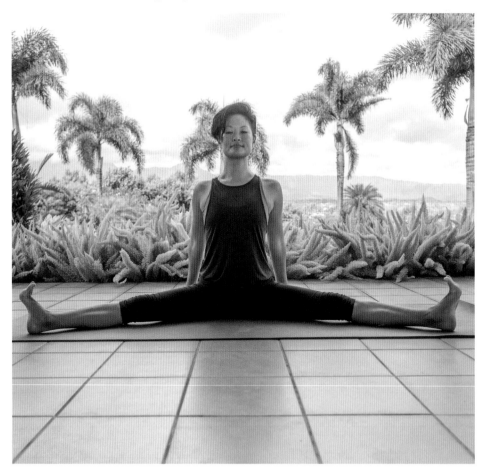

RECLINED HAND TO BIG TOE POSE

This supine version of standing hand to big toe pose supports the spine to allow for deeper lengthening of the back body and hamstrings. *Supta padangusthasana*, reclined hand to big toe pose, increases the rooting of the thigh bone on the bottom leg to lengthen the hip flexors and iliopsoas and help relieve back pain. Begin by lying on your back with your knees bent, feet hip distance apart. Press your feet, hips, ribs, shoulders, and back of the head into the earth to activate the natural curves of the spine. Bring your right knee to your chest and either hold onto the big toe with your right fingers or use a strap around the sole of the foot. Extend the right leg up toward the sky and stretch your left leg out on the ground, rooting down through the back of the leg. Take five to eight breaths here, keeping your shoulders rooting down and your left hand on top of the left thigh. Release back to active recovery pose (bridge prep) between sides.

Tips: Keep the knee of the lifted leg bent as you begin to work with this pose for as long as you need to. If it is challenging to keep the shoulders and head down, place a folded blanket under the back of the head for more comfort and ease.

Possible risks: Hamstrings and neck.

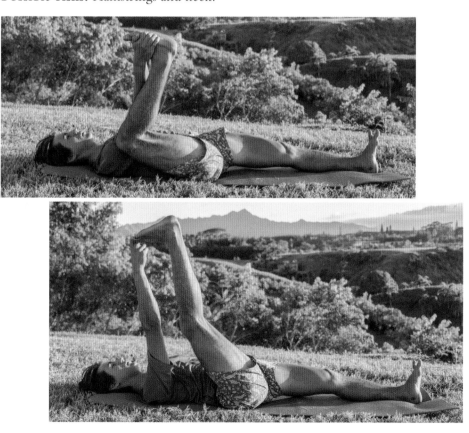

HAPPY BABY POSE

Ananda balasana, happy baby pose, is another supine deep forward fold that lengthens the inner thighs as well as the hamstrings, glutes, and back. Begin by lying on your back with your knees toward your chest. Take a few deep breaths here, hugging the knees in with your hands on your shins to lengthen the back and bring the thighs closer to the torso. Then take the knees apart, extend them to a 90-degree angle, and flex the feet so the soles face the sky. Reach your arms inside of the legs and take hold of your ankles or the outside of your feet, drawing the knees down toward the floor. Take five to eight breaths here, keeping your hips down, your shoulders grounding, and the back of the neck long.

Tips: Rocking from side to side in this posture helps massage the low back and calm the nervous system to deepen into the posture. You may also try this pose one leg at a time to begin to open the hips and back more deeply. Then try both legs at the same time.

Possible risks: Hamstrings, hips, low back, and neck.

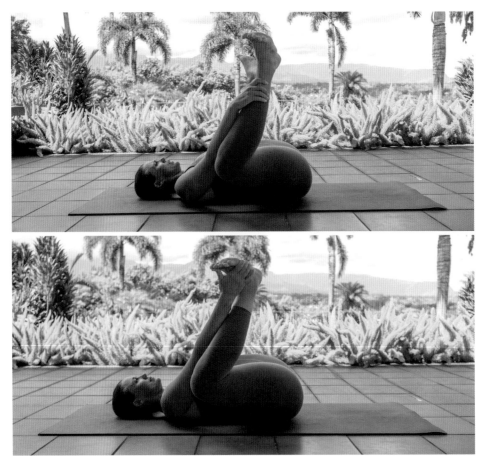

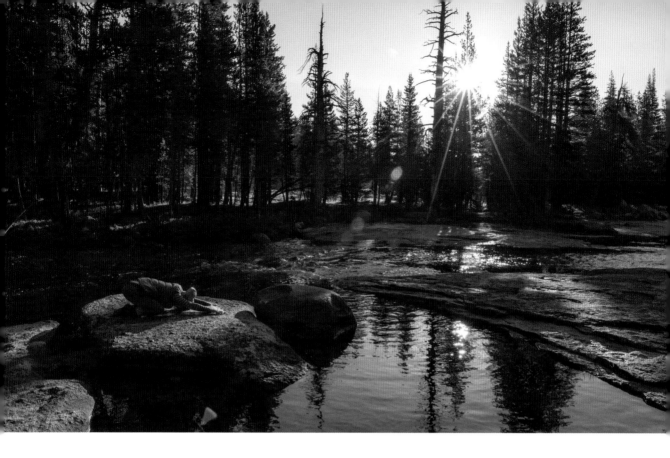

INVERSIONS AND SEMI-INVERSIONS

This class of postures is known for improving circulation and reversing the effects of gravity. Technically, inversions and semi- or half inversions are postures where the pelvis and heart are above the head. Ideally these postures can be held for 5 minutes or more for the greatest benefits. They do require strength and mobility in the shoulders, core, hips, and legs, so they are considered more advanced postures to work toward. Downward facing dog and dolphin poses are accessible inversions that build strength and mobility for the more challenging postures. Inversions are typically done at the end of a practice when the body is fully prepared.

A note for menstruating women: Traditionally it is recommended for women to avoid inversions during at least the first few days of their cycle. There has been much discussion about this recommendation over the years, without definitive consensus. It really depends on the woman and her unique personal experience. Many women who have heavy periods have reported that inverting helps relieve discomfort and slow the cycles. Other women who have regular inverting practices and lighter cycles just invert for much shorter amounts of time during the first few days. Still other women have no desire to invert at all during their cycle. The point is, you know your body and cycles—do what feels most honoring for you.

DOLPHIN POSE

This posture has emerged from the preparation of a more challenging inversion, forearm stand pose. Dolphin pose, *ardha pincha mayurasana*, is more accessible and helps build the strength, stability, and mobility required for forearm stand pose. It has many of the same benefits as downward facing dog yet with deeper shoulder opening and core strength. Begin in table pose on your hands and knees with toes tucked. Bring your forearms down to the ground with the elbows under the shoulders and shoulder width apart. Clasp your hands together and press the outer edge of your hands or keep the forearms parallel and palms grounded. Press the forearms down firmly, drawing the shoulders away from the ears and broadening the collarbones. On an inhalation, begin straightening the legs to lift your knees, hips, and back up. Press through your feet, engage your core, and root down through the arms. Let your neck relax so your crown reaches toward the floor. Stay for five to eight breaths, staying engaged as you begin to walk the feet in closer to the elbows. Release to child's pose when complete.

As this pose becomes more comfortable with your hands clasped together, begin to work with a block between your hands. This version deepens the shoulder opening and stabilizing work. Squeeze the block with your hands while simultaneously squeezing your elbows in toward the block.

Tips: This pose requires strong shoulder engagement as well as core strength and long, supple hamstrings. If hamstring tightness is an obstacle, bend your knees and widen your feet. If your shoulders are stiff and your low ribs pop out, focus on integrating the core more by drawing your front ribs down toward the top of the pelvis while pressing the shoulders down. This strengthens the core and lengthens the shoulder muscles.

Possible risks: Hamstrings, low back, shoulders, and neck.

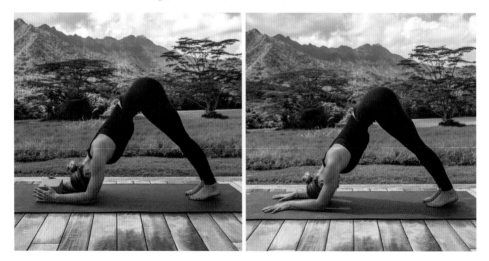

CANDLESTICK POSE

Viparitha karani, often called candlestick pose, is another fairly accessible and relaxing inversion that can be held for 5 minutes or so to help reduce swelling and fatigue in the legs, and increase overall circulation. Begin in bridge preparation pose with the knees bent and feet flat on the ground, hip distance apart. Press your arms and shoulders down to the ground as you exhale to lift the hips upward. Keep the back of the neck long, the sternum lifting toward your chin, and inner feet grounded. Place a block under your pelvis at a height that feels comfortable for you. Your weight will be on your shoulders, the back of your head, and the block with the spine at a 45-degree angle rather than your spine being perpendicular to the ground. Press into the back of the arms and head as you lift one knee at a time toward the chest, feet off the ground. Extend through your legs, engaging your glutes and core as you lift the lower body upward. Stay for as long as you can maintain the integrity of the pose, about 3 to 10 minutes.

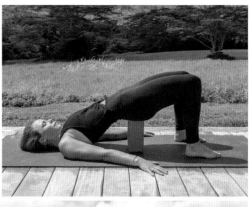

Tips: Try having the block at the lowest level first until you are comfortable with this posture. You can then play with turning the block to the medium or highest height if that feels comfortable to you.

Possible risks: Neck, wrists, and low back.

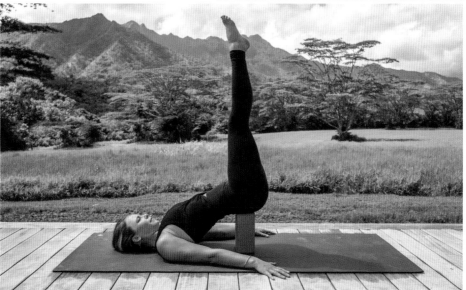

HANDSTAND

Urdhva mukha virkshasana, upward facing tree or handstand pose, is a challenging inversion that builds strength in the legs, core, shoulders, and arms. It is not a pose most people can hold for long periods but is classified as an inversion because it meets all the other requirements. This posture can help stabilize the core and shoulder girdle, which is helpful for paddlers, climbers, and anyone who is ready to face the fears of being upside down, and build strength in the upper body. Practicing close to a wall of some kind or with the help of a friend helps reduce the fear of falling over and helps build enough comfort and experience in the pose to move away from the wall.

Begin in downward facing dog pose with the hands about a foot away from a wall or your friend's foot. Keeping your hands firmly rooting down and shoulders broad, move your chest forward so your shoulders are over your wrists. Take a step forward with one foot in a short lunge pose. Lift the opposite leg up, keeping it straight and internally rotating. If a friend is helping you, he or she should hold onto the outer hips lightly. Pushing down through your hands with straight arms, push off your lunging leg on an inhalation to move your hips over your shoulders toward the wall or your friend. Lift both legs up into the support of the wall or your friend. Look down toward your hands, and draw your belly and front ribs in as you extend up through your hips and legs. Slowly start to move one foot then the other away from the wall, playing with finding your balance as you breathe. Come down into standing forward fold to release and try again.

Tips: Practicing dolphin pose helps build the stability and mobility in the shoulders required for this pose. Holding plank pose for 30 to 60 seconds or more is a great way to strengthen the core for handstands as well.

Possible risks: Wrists, shoulders, and low back.

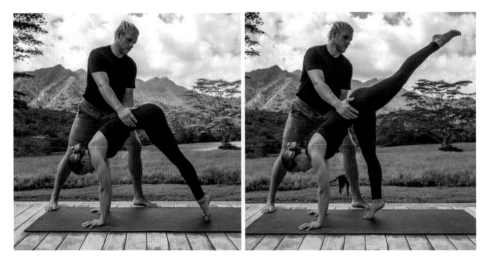

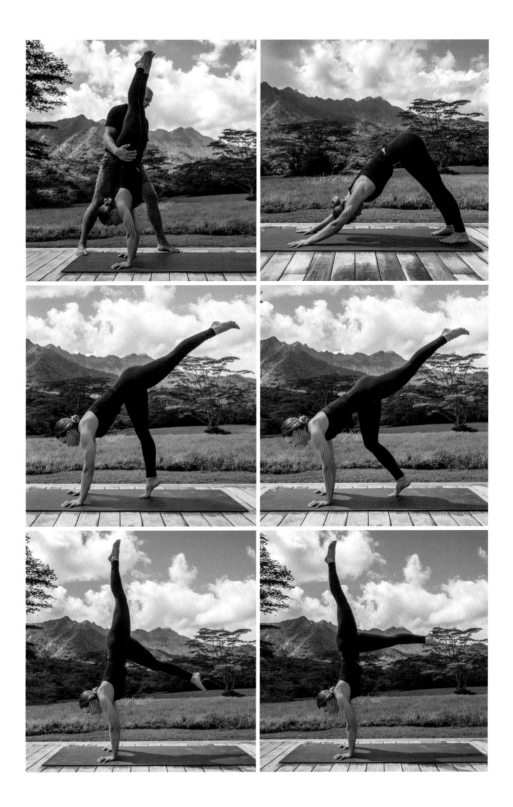

SHOULDERSTAND

This posture builds upon bridge pose and *viparitha karani* (candlestick pose) with the weight of the body supported on the upper arms, shoulders, and the back of the head. *Salamba sarvangasana*, shoulderstand, builds leg, core, and shoulder strength and creates a strong flexion of the neck. Begin in bridge preparation pose with the arms pressing down. Draw your knees toward the forehead, lifting the feet and hips off the ground. Place your hands on the back of the lower ribs as high as you can with ease. Pressing the back of your head and shoulders down, extend up through your core, hips, and legs, pointing your feet toward the sky. Stay for as long as you can maintain the lift of the torso and legs and maintain integrity in the neck and shoulders. Gaze toward the toes.

Tips: Root the back of the upper arms and elbows down firmly, lengthen your breath, and soften your gaze up toward your toes.

Possible risks: Neck, shoulders, and low back.

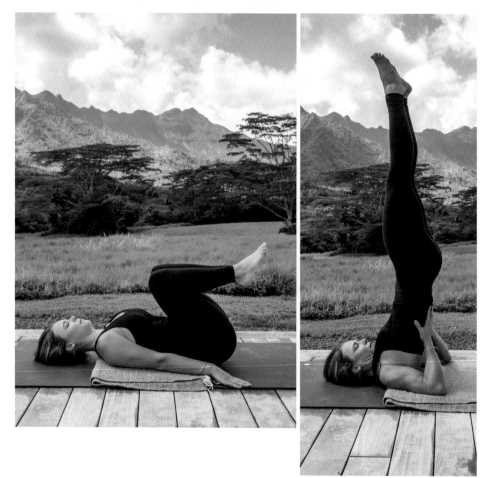

PLOW POSE

Halasana, plow pose, is an inverted forward fold much like seated staff pose with deep upper back lengthening. Begin by lying on your back with your palms pressing down into the ground. Bring your knees to your chest and extend your legs straight up as you lift your pelvis off the ground, then reach your toes toward the floor behind your head. Extend through your core and up through your hips as you draw your shoulder blades closer together on your back and interlace your fingers, rooting the arms down. Lengthen the back of your neck as the chest comes closer to the chin, and press the center of the back of the head down as you reach through your legs. Stay for ten to twenty breaths before releasing.

Tips: If your toes do not touch the ground, place a block or blanket on the ground beyond the head before entering the pose. If clasping your fingers is challenging, keep your arms at your sides, pressing your palms down and squeezing your shoulder blades together.

Possible risks: Neck, low back, hamstrings, and shoulders.

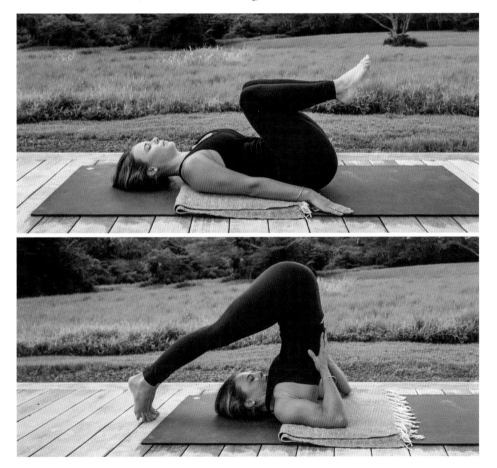

HEADSTAND

For the purposes of this book we will look at *salamba sirsasana one*, headstand, with the hands clasped together and forearms on the earth. This posture builds shoulder and neck stability and strengthens the core, hips, and legs. There is a slight pressure on the top of the head, the crown, that is said to help center and calm the mind while flushing oxygenated blood into the brain. Begin in table pose, then bring your forearms to the ground, elbows directly under the shoulders, and clasp the hands together. Press the flat part of the top of your head down on the ground just in front of your clasped hands and draw your shoulders away from your ears by rooting down through the forearms. Lift the knees and walk the feet forward toward your head until your hips are over your shoulders. Maintain the press through the top of your head and arms as you inhale and use your core to draw the knees to your chest, lifting the feet off the ground. Avoid jumping or hopping the legs up. Once you find your balance, extend through your legs, engaging through your core, hips, and legs. Take ten to twenty breaths here, then return to child's pose to rest.

Tips: Practicing dolphin pose helps you prepare for headstand. Start practicing headstand next to a wall to reduce the fear and possibility of falling over. Take your time at the wall. To begin to get comfortable with your weight on your forearms and top of the head, practice keeping the knees in a tucked position and taking ten to twenty breaths there before you work on extending your legs. This will help stabilize the core, improve balance, and get you comfortable with the mechanics. Headstand can take years of practice for some people to become comfortable and confident in it. Be patient and persistent.

Possible risks: Neck, shoulders, and low back.

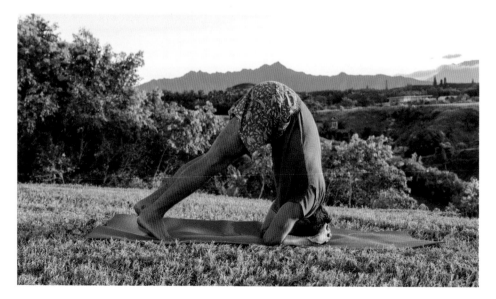

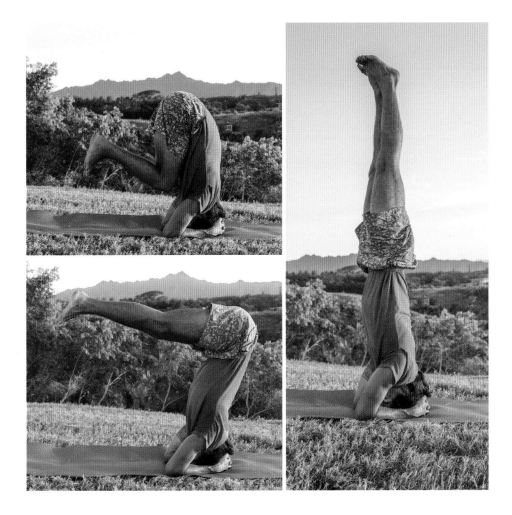

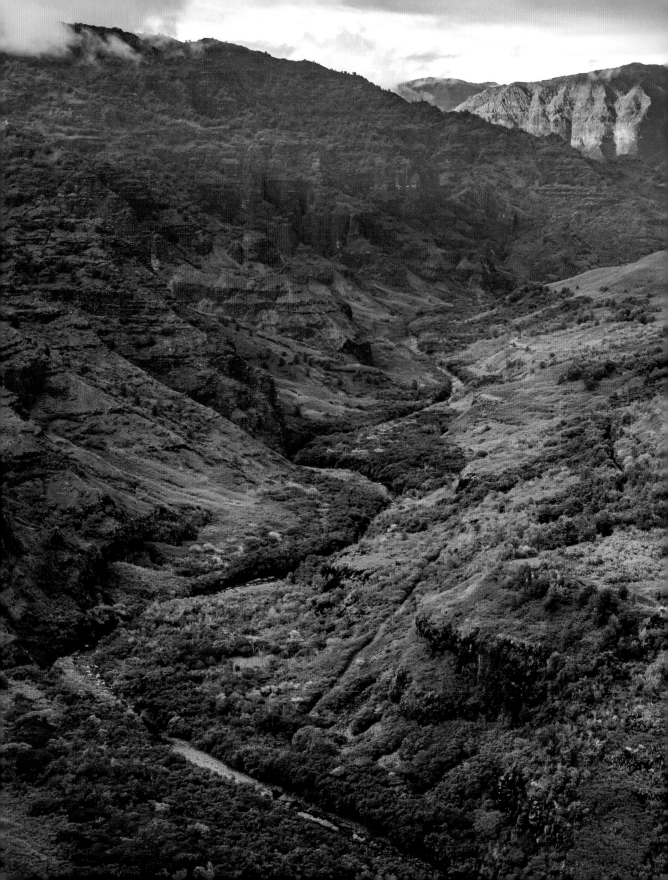

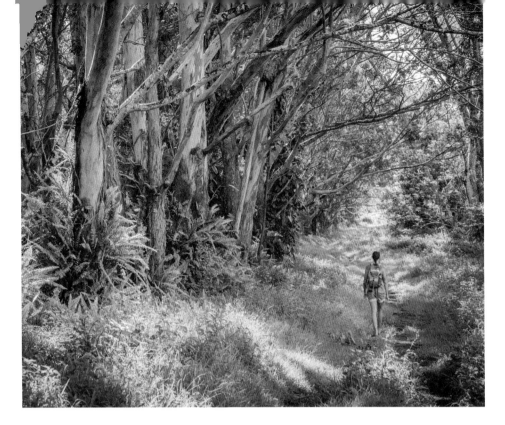

CHAPTER 6

YOGA FOR HIKING

A walk in nature walks the soul back home.
—MARY DAVIS

IT WAS MY TIME IN NEPAL that really opened up the world of hiking to me. On a four-day backpacking trip through the Annapurna region of the Himalayas, I experienced that sublime feeling of oneness that is the goal of both yoga and out-door adventure. Heart pounding, feet aching, hiking through the rhododendron forest, I emerged to see the river far below and the snowy peaks ahead, and my heart burst open. I was hooked on hiking. Trails are definitely my happy place and bring me to that pure state of *sat-chit-ananda* (truth–consciousness–bliss) that the texts of yoga speak of as the highest state of being. Combining hiking with the practices of yoga out in the wild and sharing it with others is one of the greatest gifts of my life. My daily practice enables me to get out on the trail and into nature with far more strength, grace, respect, and awareness. It also helps me recover from a long day of hiking far faster, so I can enjoy my surroundings and the next day even more.

GETTING TRAIL READY

One of the greatest traits of the human species is the ability to walk upright, or *bipedalism*. The earliest evidence of this evolutionary feat comes from a 4.4-million-year-old hominid fossil. Walking on two feet made early hominids more intimidating to predators and freed their hands to carry things and make tools. Undoubtedly, walking is part of what makes us human. In an industrialized world, though, it's less and less a part of everyday life. Traditional nomadic hunter-gatherer populations walked an average of 7 miles per day. Americans take 5,117 steps a day—or around 2.5 miles. That's significantly less than our peers in Western Australia (9,695 steps a day), Switzerland (9,650), and Japan (7,168). Around the globe, though, we simply walk less and less. Most of us can't, practically speaking, walk 7 miles every day. That's all the more reason to step out of your routine and onto the trail a little more often.

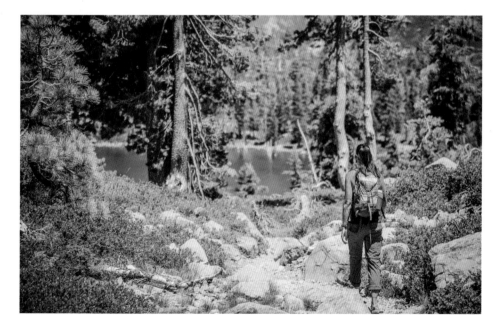

"   AS WE LEAVE URBAN AREAS AND HEAD INTO NATURE, TRAIL TERRAIN WILL VARY AND CHALLENGE OUR HABITUAL MOVEMENT PATTERNS, ALLOWING FOR STRENGTH-BUILDING BUT ALSO INVARIABLY SHOWING US OUR WEAK SPOTS."

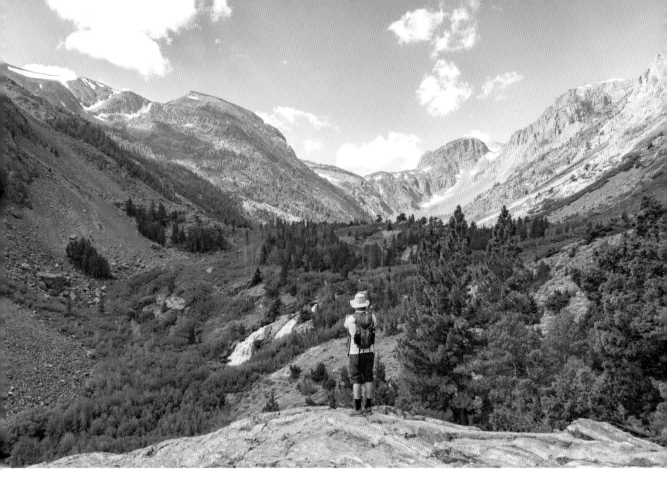

Walking has endless health benefits. Just 30 minutes a day aids in maintaining healthy weight, improves mood, enhances balance and coordination, and strengthens muscles and bones. The more you walk the greater the health benefits, based on Mayo Clinic findings. As we get out into nature for walking and hiking on more varied terrain, the benefits increase even more. A study done by the European Centre for Environment and Human Health at the University of Exeter in the UK found that approximately 2 hours per week spent in nature has an overwhelming positive impact on health. Some of these benefits include lower blood pressure and stress hormone levels, calmer nervous system, strengthened immune function, increased self-esteem, improved mood, and reduced anxiety. In times of stress, getting out into nature for a walk or hike has tremendous power to shift our mental, emotional, and physical response to what in our modern times can often feel like a world of constant stress. Most of us know the power of nature: We crave time outside because it helps us to feel better whether we know why or not.

Humans evolved to move in dynamic and diverse ways, but as our bodies have gotten used to flat ground and modern furniture, our natural movement patterns have withered. Many of us sit too long and move in limited ways. Walking on

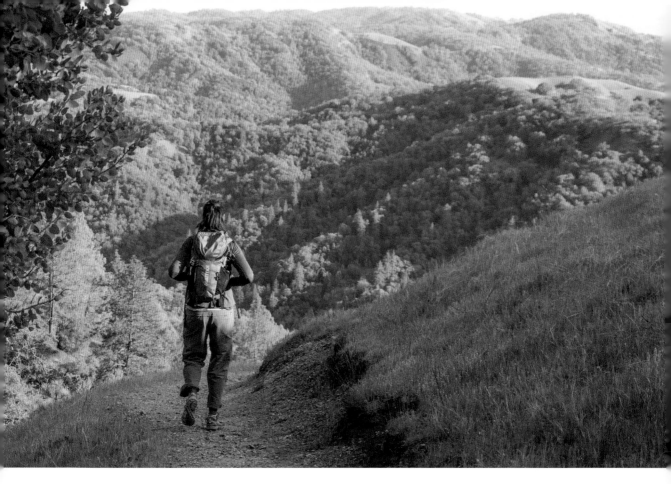

pavement, within buildings, on flat surfaces, and in shoes designed for looks (not function) trains our bodies in certain movements, leaving out all others. Squatting, getting up and down off the floor without the use of our hands, carrying and pulling heavy things, and climbing are all part of our human capacity. Modern conveniences have removed most of these daily movements, so we have to seek them out now. As we leave urban areas and head into nature, trail terrain will vary and challenge our habitual movement patterns, allowing for strength-building but also invariably showing us our weak spots. Practicing yoga builds body awareness and postural balance. As we dive into the demands of hiking in this chapter, we will explore the endless ways yoga can not only reintroduce natural human movements but also help along the trail.

Walking puts weight on your heels and stretches the arches and Achilles tendons (the base of the calf muscles that connect to the heel). If you have worn shoes with a heel, even an inch or so, for many years, as most of us have, your foot and ankle mobility may be limited. Begin by noticing how you walk, what part of your foot hits the ground first. What's the second area of contact? Where is the last point of contact before your foot lifts again?

As the youngest in my family, I was often chasing after my brothers and cousins and had plenty of skinned knees and crashes. Injuries led to misalignments and eventually limited my range of motion, decreased my energy, and increased my propensity for further injury. Twisted ankles and sore knees became the norm and kept me from getting deeper into nature. As I began hiking more and falling in love with trail life, I found it necessary to address these old structural imbalances. Stretching helped, but it was developing a daily yoga practice that increased my overall strength, stability, and mobility to get outdoors more often. After years of barefoot practice, twisted ankles no longer threaten my adventures. Now my body is strong enough to withstand rugged trails, and my practice helps me minimize or avoid injuries. My enjoyment and love of hiking has grown exponentially as old patterns have shifted. I no longer dread the pain and fatigue of time on the trail, but instead seek out longer hikes and more challenging terrain. Meditation, breathing practices, and *asana* have helped me to focus, be present in the moment, and engage with my surroundings in new ways—all while enjoying the journey.

Hiking is often the entry point for many other outdoor sports, leading us literally down the path to greater connection with nature. So what are the biggest demands on the body when hiking? Foot and ankle mobility and strength, knee strain, leg and hip strength, low back health, core strength, and shoulder and neck health all factor into a happy, healthy hike. Healthy breathing patterns and mental awareness are also key to enjoying and staying safe on and off the trail. Let's take a closer look at each area.

ANATOMY OF HIKING

Feet/Ankles

Each foot has twenty-six bones, thirty-three muscles, thirty-one joints, and over one hundred ligaments. Two longitudinal arches and one transverse arch form the structure of each foot. The weight and movement of the whole body is built on this framework, from the arches through the pelvis and up to the head and neck.

Your feet absorb feedback with every step and translate information to the rest of your body. Slight imbalances in the foot strike can lead to musculoskeletal strain in asymmetrical patterns through the fascia (connective tissue), muscles, and nervous system. Begin to notice how you walk and how you stand. Most of us have the habit of standing on one foot more than the other or standing with our weight unevenly distributed between the feet. Do your feet turn out or perhaps in? Maybe one of your feet turns just a bit more than the other. Pay attention to how your weight is distributed on each foot.

TRY THIS

With bare feet, walk in place with your eyes closed for 10 to 20 seconds, then stop. Open your eyes and look down at your feet. Feel into them; notice how your feet are placed and where the weight feels heavier or lighter. If they are not already, try to bring your feet parallel so your knees face forward. Next, shift your weight so it is more evenly distributed between your left and right foot, from front to back and side to side. Since the feet are the primary foundation for the whole body, balancing weight more evenly helps align the spine and center of gravity. Balance is improved as well as mobility all the way up the body.

Trails offer much more diverse terrain than the average person's feet and ankles are used to. Hiking uphill requires the ankle to bend to a more acute degree (dorsiflexion) than in everyday life. Even walking up flights of stairs or training on a stair climber keeps the feet fairly flat. When we walk on uneven surfaces uphill, we can experience strain and tenderness in the feet, Achilles tendon, calves, knees, and low back. Downhill hiking creates plantar flexion, meaning you're basically walking on tiptoe, stretching the front of your ankle joint as you walk downhill. That's not an angle where our bodies are generally prepared to be strong. It can lead to soreness in the ankle, the front of the shin muscles, the knee joint, and again the low back. Even on relatively level terrain, the feet are constantly turning in (inversion) or out (eversion) to get over rocks and forest debris, challenging the ankles. And all that is just when day hiking. Any weight in your pack will compound the impact of every step. Carrying everything you need for a week in the wilderness on your back, then challenging your stamina at an increased range of motion ups the risk of rolling or spraining your ankle.

All the time we spend in ill-fitting shoes limits strength and mobility in the feet. As you begin to stretch and demand more of your feet, they will get stronger and more supple, but it takes time. The practice of yoga can both rehabilitate your feet and prepare them for the joys and rigors of hiking. The first step is taking off your shoes and stepping onto your mat. Practicing yoga barefoot as well as spending more of your time in general with bare feet will help open up and strengthen the feet. Stiff and high-heeled shoes limit foot sensitivity and range of motion, making hiking quite the shock to calves and feet. Lower heels and flexible shoes are gaining favor in the hiking world, allowing for more mobility and strength in the feet and lower legs, providing a greater sensitivity for changing terrain. Don't rush it, though—transition shoes over six months to a year to minimize injuries. Some people's medical conditions may require higher heels and more stable footwear on and off the trail, so always consider your body's unique demands when choosing gear. There are many postures and therapeutic practices for the feet that may still be used.

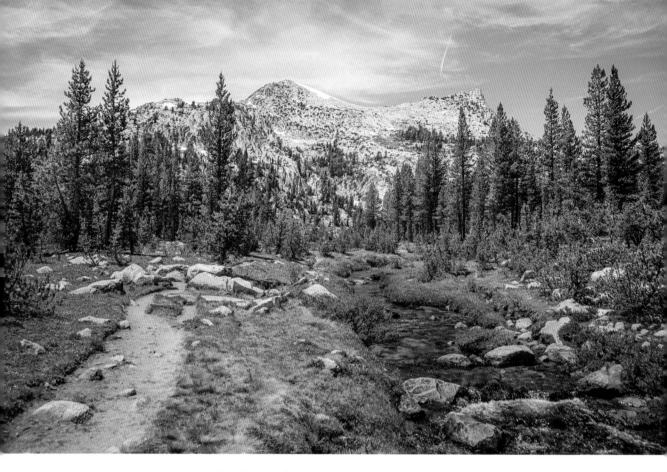

Yoga is practiced with bare feet, which helps increase the foundational awareness and work out imbalances. Simply by allowing the feet to spread and move in every direction, the muscles, tendons, and ligaments begin to change. Practicing a wide variety of postures also helps increase blood flow to the feet and ankles as well as improve nerve health, which often suffers in shoes. Barefoot practice helps wake up our feet and create better balance when walking. Spreading the toes and becoming more dexterous with our feet helps us navigate challenging terrain with greater ease and grace. In addition, a post-hike practice can relieve aching feet and reduce both swelling and soreness by releasing tension, improving circulation, and addressing foot strike imbalances.

In my late twenties I participated in daylong meditation retreats where seated meditation was broken up with walking meditation. At the time I was working waiting tables, doing environmental education for schools, and running often. During my first walking meditation, I learned how poor my balance was, how imbalanced my gait was, and how painful and tight my feet were. It was humbling and extremely informative. Walking slowly showed me how I was more weighted on the outsides of my feet, and that the weight was imbalanced from left to right. My heels struck

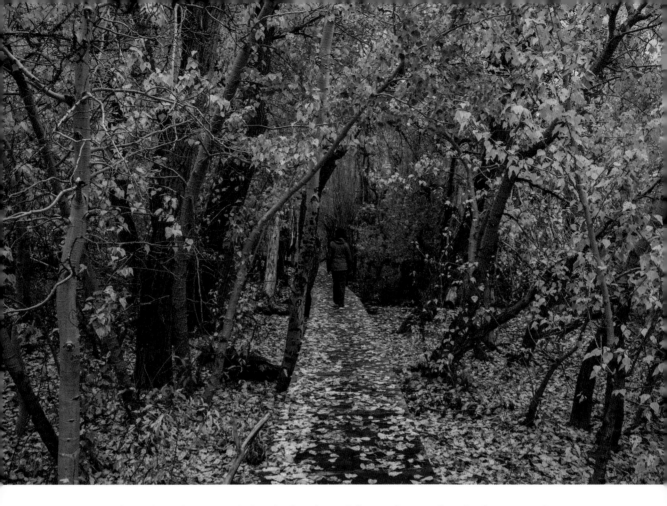

heavily and my knees tended to lock. I leaned forward at my low back too much, using momentum to carry me instead of muscle and coordination. The next time I ran, I could see these patterns clearly. When I hiked across rocks, I now understood why I felt so wobbly and unstable. So I got different shoes with lower heel lift and a wider toe box. I began rolling tennis balls under my arches and practicing specific yoga postures to improve my foot and ankle health. The next time I did a walking meditation, I noticed marked improvement in balance, ease, and flexibility.

TRY THIS

Walking meditation is a powerful way to learn about your foot strike. Find a space out in nature—a field or beach works well to give you more feedback. With bare feet, walk as slowly as possible for 10 minutes or so. Keep your eyes ahead instead of down at your feet. Pay close attention to how the weight shifts on your foot as you begin to peel one off the ground and lift it. Note which parts of your foot leave the earth first, your balance, and all the muscles involved. Note how the weight changes on your other foot as it takes your whole weight. What muscles are lifting your one leg, and what muscles are propelling you forward on the grounded foot? As you move slowly forward, at a snail's pace, notice any other shifts in your body position, such as low back and head. When the lifted foot begins to touch the ground again, note which parts hit first, second, third. Continue to walk as slow as imaginable, paying attention to the shifts in your feet, weight, and whole body as you move forward. This practice helps us notice the small movements of walking and shows us challenges we may not notice when we walk fast.

When we look closer at walking, we see that the entire body is involved. Ideally the center of the heel strikes first, then the balls of the foot, and finally, your toes bend as you push off the big toe. The calf muscles engage, and the front and sides of the shin muscles, thighs, inner thighs, hamstrings, glutes, and core all fire to move us forward. There is a twisting of the trunk as we walk that engages the shoulders and arms to swing, which helps us maintain balance as we move forward. Finally, this gentle twisting creates free flow in the shoulder girdle that allows for the head to stay fairly neutral, keeping our eyes focused on the terrain and path ahead. But it all begins with the foot strike—the way our feet land and move as we take each step. The walking meditation practice outlined above will show you which part of your foot strikes the ground first when walking. Whatever your normal pattern may be, try to land mid-heel first and then roll forward through the foot, keeping your weight centered as much as you can.

To get ready for the trail, start logging some extra walks three to four days a week. Get out onto city or state park trails whenever you can. Get proper-fitting shoes with minimal heel lift and room for your toes to spread. Begin or restart a regular yoga practice at least three times a week to increase the range of motion and stability of your ankle joints and strengthen your feet. Take your shoes off and walk barefoot around your home as much as you can.

COMMON FOOT INJURIES

Plantar fasciitis prevents many people from hiking and is one of the top injuries for hikers in general. When the fibrous tissue (plantar fascia) along the bottom of your foot that connects your heel bone to your toes becomes inflamed, it creates intense pain while walking. Stretching your feet and using a tennis ball for foot massage is the best way to treat and prevent this injury, along with investing in shoes that fit properly. With bare feet, place one foot on top of a tennis ball. Roll the ball along the sole of the foot including the arches and under the balls of the toes for 30 seconds or so. Next, stand with the ball under the mounds of the toes and press your weight into it for 30 seconds. Switch the ball to the arch and press for another 30 seconds or so. Lastly, place the ball under your heel and press firmly for five deep breaths. Switch to the other foot and repeat. Repeat a few times daily while in acute pain and daily as needed.

Heel spurs are bony growths on the heel that make each step painful. This often compromises foot strike as you try to avoid the painful area. Heel spurs often occur along with plantar fasciitis, caused by the muscle and ligament strain pulling on the bottom of the foot. Again, stretching, practicing yoga, and massage are good ways to prevent and treat heel spurs, although medical treatment may be necessary.

Blisters—we've all had them. Ill-fitting shoes or socks are often the culprit, but blisters can develop over enough miles even with the best gear. Spots on our feet that rub against a shoe, step after step, mile after mile, will blister and skin can tear away. These are painful and can also lead to changes in our gait pattern to avoid the pain. Take the time to get good-fitting shoes and break them in before a hike, and wear good socks. Changing your socks daily and keeping your feet dry also helps prevent blisters. The body awareness that yoga builds helps us be more alert to rubbing and the beginning of blister pain. Address these spots early with extra cushioning using moleskin or socks.

Bunions are another painful foot issue that may keep people from walking and hiking. Caused by narrow shoes and excessive pressure on your big toe joint when you walk, a bunion is a lump of bone or tissue on the side of your big toe joint that can cause the joint to misalign and rotate, creating pain with each step. Practicing yoga, walking barefoot, massage, and shoes with plenty of room in the toe box can help reduce the onset of bunions and help alleviate pain.

Knees

One quarter of American adults suffer from knee pain. My own knee injuries began in 1997 during my first trip to Nepal. I was in a motorbike accident and tore one of the ligaments in my knee. Since surgery was not an option, I elevated and iced my knee over the next week or so and limited movements that aggravated it. Over the next few years, as I logged more miles hiking and running, my knees were always my limiting factor. It was my yoga practice that created the balance, strength, and mobility in my lower body that I needed to heal my knees. Rehabilitating my knees was a large motivation for me to create a daily, ongoing practice that has since allowed me to log many miles and adventure to incredible places.

As a hinge joint, the knee is designed to flex or extend. It can tolerate very little twisting or lateral movement without injury. While this works fine in our flat, civilized world, trails present a challenge. The key to healthy knees begins with the feet and ankles. As we just learned, foot and ankle issues will affect everything above them and can create misalignment in the knees, hips, and low back. Tight calves and hamstrings, thigh muscles, hip flexors, or posterior hips will create uneven stress on the knee joint. When the calf muscles are tight and weak from underuse, the strain will usually fall on the feet, then the front of the knee joint. Hamstring tension creates a pulling on the outer knee and back of the knee, sometimes leading to Baker's cyst (swelling in the popliteal space, the space behind the knee, also known as a popliteal cyst) or hyperextension (straightening the knee joint beyond normal range of motion, causing swelling and pain). Quadriceps and hip flexor dominance will typically strain the inner knee and hip.

A well-rounded yoga practice not only helps improve foot and ankle health, but also can help stabilize the knees. The key is to begin with simple postures and slowly progress to more weight-bearing postures. Work the feet and hips especially. The hike sequences below include some of the more common postures to help rehabilitate or prepare the knees.

Hips

As our ancestors became bipedal, the shape of the low back and pelvis (the two hip bones, sacrum, and coccyx) began to change. In order to carry the weight of the upper body in a vertical position, humans developed a larger pelvic girdle (the hip bone and sacrum) and longer iliopsoas muscles (the biggest hip flexor muscles that run from the anterior superior lumbar spine to the inner upper thigh bone). As the seat of the spine, the pelvis carries a great deal of weight, load, and stress. The pelvis is made up of three bones, the ilium, ischium, and pubic bones, which fuse in childhood. The iliosacral joints are on either side of the sacrum, forming the keystone of the low back. The hip joint is a ball-and-socket joint where the femur (thigh bone) meets the pelvis.

Hips are designed to move in just about every direction—in flexion, extension, adduction, abduction, medial rotation, and lateral rotation. All of these movements affect the entirety of the body. These actions typically happen at the hip joint, though the pelvis does move forward and backward in anteversion (anterior tilt) and retroversion (posterior tilt). Many people experience torsion (rotation) on one side of the iliosacral joint. This occurs when one ilium is rotated, displacing the sacroiliac joint on that side. This torsion can be very painful, but it can also be present with no symptoms and can still cause muscle imbalances downward through the foot and upward through the spine. Any imbalances make themselves known during repetitive motion such as long-distance hiking.

Since the pelvis has so many attachment sites for muscles that move in every direction, it is easy to see how imbalances and misalignment can lead to injuries or chronic pain in the hips and low back. Walking trails, especially uphill, requires slight forward flexion of the trunk at the hips. Notice how you lean forward slightly while hiking, and how much greater that lean is when carrying a pack. The key is to both allow this forward motion and balance it through the legs, core, and head position. Drive the force downward through the hips, hamstrings, calves, and feet

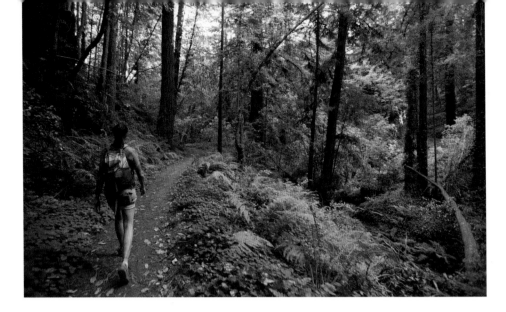

while stabilizing the core and extending through the crown of the head. That sounds like a lot to remember all at once, but it's exactly what we practice in yoga postures such as mountain pose.

Core/Torso

While your legs and feet carry you along the trail, it's your core (including your low back) that translates that movement upward through the body. A strong core goes a long way in helping the shoulders and back, saving energy, effort, and soreness. Stabilizing your core and entire torso from front, back, and sides will go a long way to reduce injuries and exhaustion.

So, what is the core exactly? Technically it extends from the shoulders to the pelvis including layers of superficial muscles, deep stabilizing muscles, and the muscles of the shoulders and hips. Over the years our understanding and definition of the core has evolved. Once thought of as the abdominal muscles (rectus abdominis, internal and external obliques), the anatomical core is now understood to include the abdominal muscles, iliopsoas, pelvic floor muscles, deep gluteal muscles and quadratus lumborum, and erector spinae on the back of the body.

Training your core doesn't just mean crunches and leg lifts. While these actions can engage the superficial abdominal muscles listed above, they do not target the deeper intrinsic muscles that support the spine. It is these deep core muscles that help support and move the lower thoracic and lumbar spine and pelvis. These muscles are often poorly developed in our modern world, leading to back pain and spinal instability. With full yogic breathing you can learn to recruit the deepest muscles and create a strong, supple, and efficient core. The anatomy of breathing and detailed practices can be found in the anatomy and alignment chapters.

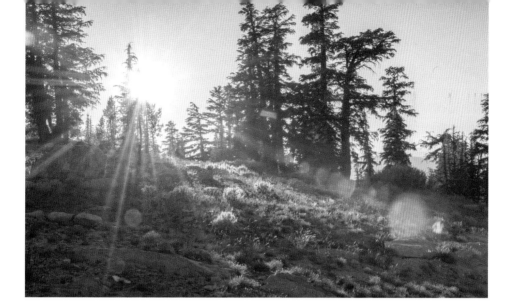

Practicing yoga will help improve the overall health of your trunk. Engage *oujaii* breathing throughout your yoga practice to recruit your core muscles, and watch your posture throughout the day. Add long holds in certain postures such as plank, side plank, crow pose, boat pose, and mountain pose to increase muscle endurance, and you will soon be ready for a long through hike. Work core postures into your weekly practice, a little more or longer each time. Unlike the bigger muscles of the body such as quads or shoulders, the abdominal muscles can be trained daily. Conscious breathing will go a long way to support you from the inside out by retraining the deepest muscles along the spine.

Upper Body

The sternum, or breastbone, is the only place where the shoulder girdle attaches to the trunk. While this allows the shoulders to have greater range of motion, they are far more likely to be injured through repetitive strain or acute injury such as a dislocation. Creating balance between mobility and strength is key. With a pack on your back, your shoulders will tend to round forward, tightening your pectorals and straining your neck. In addition, lifting your pack may aggravate wrists, elbows, and low back. The lifting and twisting motion will challenge any imbalances in the body. Focusing on opening the chest while strengthening the back and arms will help reduce risk and increase the joy of the trail.

SEQUENCES FOR HIKING

Many of these postures can be done either lying down on a mat or sitting in a chair to be more accessible. Start practicing the sequences three times a week to get familiar with them and begin to prepare yourself for your adventures.

Training Sequence

This builds strength, mobility, balance, core integrity, and overall body awareness. Practice this sequence three times a week for four to six weeks before a big hiking trip.

(1) Reclined centering with deep breaths (3–5 minutes)

(2) Reclined knees to chest pose

(3) Wind relieving pose

(4) Reclined twist

(5) Leg lifts

(6) Bridge press

(7) Cat/cow poses

(8) Table twists

(9) Locust pose

(10) High plank pose

(11) Sun salutations A and B (see page 70)

(12) Warrior one pose to warrior three pose

(13) Warrior two pose to reverse warrior pose

(14) Side angle pose to half moon pose

(15) Triangle pose to half moon variations

(16) Wide legged forward fold

(17) *Skandasana*

(18) Pyramid pose

(19) Revolved triangle pose variations

(20) Tree pose

(21) Standing pigeon pose

(22) Hand to big toe pose variations

(23) Crow pose variations

(24) Locust pose variations

(25) Bow pose

(26) Simple seated twist

(27) Head to knee pose variations

(28) Bridge/wheel pose

(29) Reclined twist

(30) Happy baby pose

(31) Shoulderstand variation

(32) Headstand variation

(33) *Nadi shodhana* (10 rounds)

(34) Corpse pose

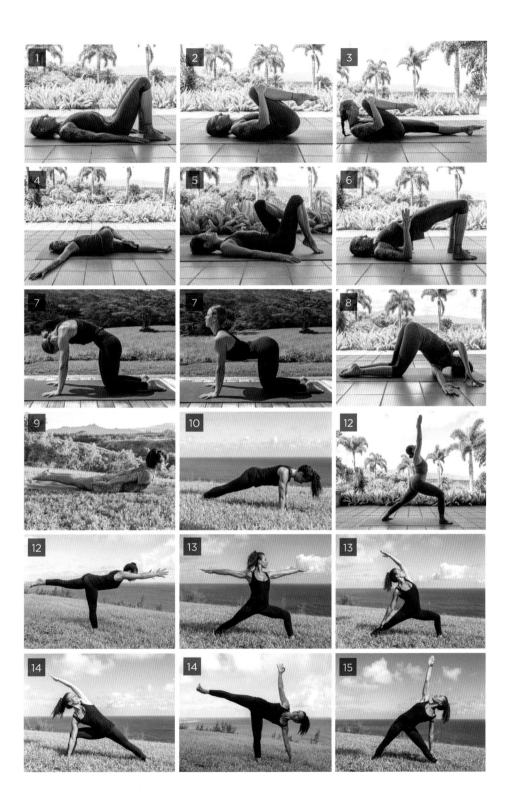

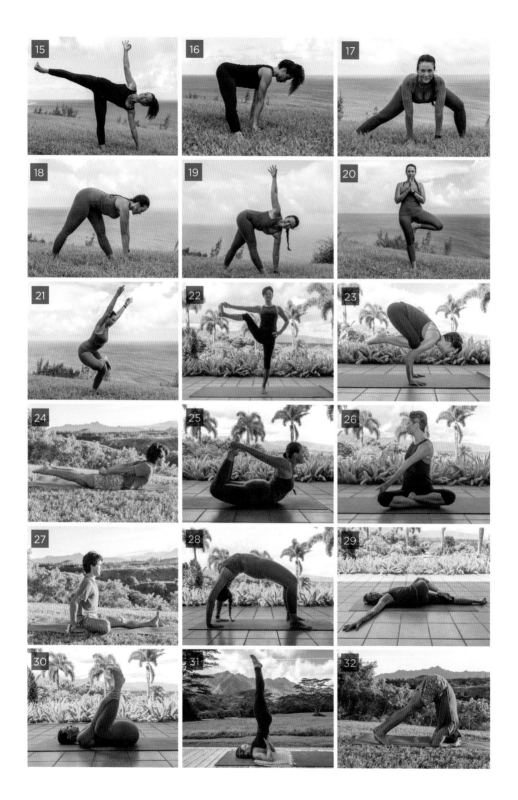

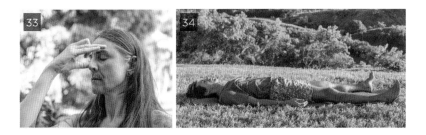

Pre-hike Sequence

This practice gets you warmed up and ready for the trail. Practice it at the trailhead (be mindful to stay out of the way of other hikers).

(1) Joint rotations (see pages 51–53)
(2) Upward salute pose
(3) Forward fold
(4) Low lunge pose
(5) Downward facing dog pose
(6) Upward facing dog pose
(7) Warrior two pose
(8) Side angle pose
(9) Forward fold
(10) Warrior three pose
(11) Dancer pose
(12) Standing pigeon pose
(13) Tree pose
(14) Standing crescent pose

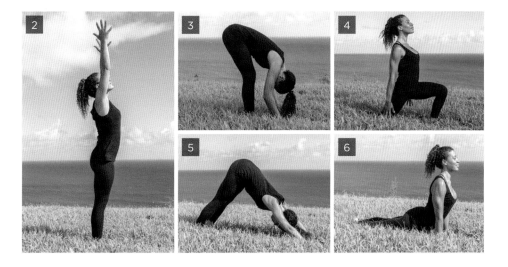

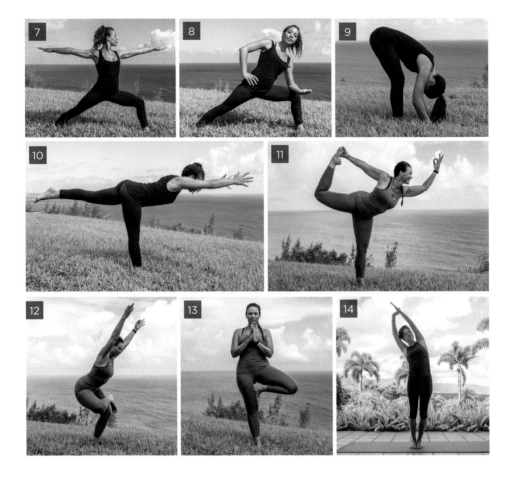

Mid-hike Sequence

This sequence is great during a break on a long hike to revive your legs, back, and upper body. Make sure you find a nice spot off the path.

(1) Upward salute pose
(2) Wide legged forward fold
(3) Low lunge pose
(4) Downward facing dog pose
(5) Upward facing dog pose
(6) Twisted thigh stretch
(7) Standing knee to chest pose
(8) Dancer pose
(9) Pyramid pose
(10) Wide legged forward fold
(11) Upward salute pose

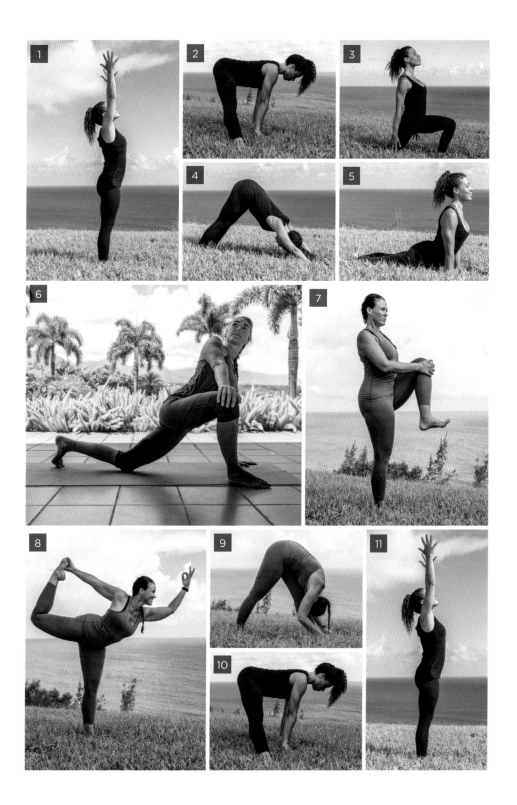

Post-hike Sequence

After a long hike this sequence will unwind all the hardworking muscles, restore energy, and improve recovery time. Find a big boulder or a good tree to help with some of the poses if you like.

(1) Downward facing dog pose
(2) Standing forward fold
(3) Low lunge pose
(4) Runner's stretch
(5) Twisted thigh stretch
(6) Standing pigeon pose
(7) Hand to big toe pose variations
(8) Dancer pose
(9) Downward facing dog pose
(10) Garland pose
(11) Simple seated twist
(12) Head to knee pose
(13) Seated forward fold
(14) Cobbler's pose
(15) *Nadi shodhana* (10 rounds)
(16) Meditation

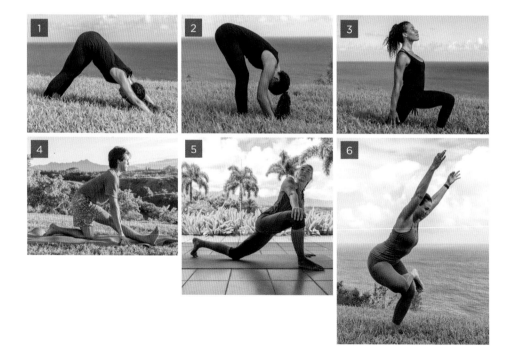

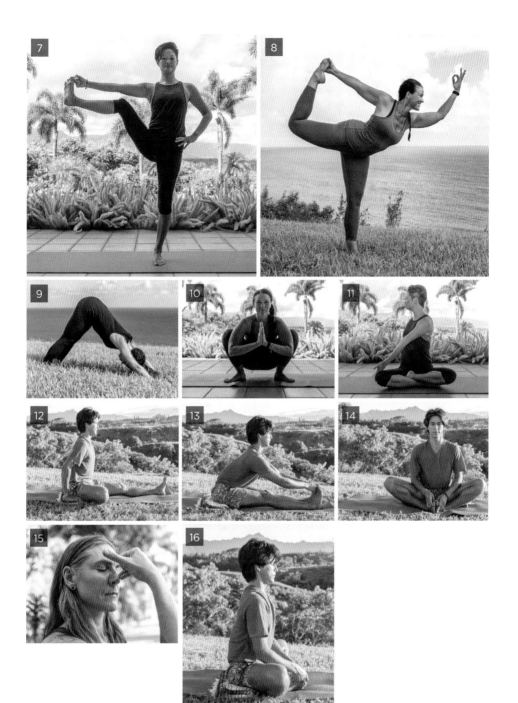

YOGI INSIGHT

HEATHER SULLIVAN

co-founder and executive director Balanced Rock Foundation, E-RYT 500
yoga instructor, founder Yosemite Healing Arts, writer; Yosemite, CA.

What about hiking drew you in?
In high school I was a three sport athlete and was used to hard work. When I started hiking in college, it was so much easier, and getting to the top of mountains and seeing big expansive views was incredible. There is something powerful about getting that big perspective and understanding the surrounding topography. It helps me see where I am in the world and how it all connects on the land and within myself.

What other outdoor sports do you love?
I spend a lot of my life outdoors, so it depends on the season. I ski in the winter, river board in the spring, climb when I can. Hiking is a constant—it takes me out to climb, up the slopes, to the river, and up into the cold alpine lakes.

How does yoga support your outdoor sports?
It has changed over my life. At first I was really into the strong physical practice and loved the discipline; I was used to it. As I've learned more of the yoga philosophy, *pranayama*, and meditation, my practice changed to more breath and meditation. If I can't get a full practice in, I meditate and do *pranayama* because it translates as more energy throughout my days. It's a bonus if I get the sun salutations and other things into my body because it feels so good. Physically, the more active I am in other sports, then my practice is softer, more restorative, nourishing for balance. I had to learn that.

What did you find most challenging about yoga when you first started?
Sitting, definitely. I would always skip out on *savasana* too. I was too restless. I just couldn't understand why or how I could just lie there. It took me a long time to learn stillness.

How has your yoga practice helped you during times of injury?
I've had many injuries and it's always helped me. A while back I tore a ligament in my thumb skiing and cancelled a ski trip. I went on a ten-day Vipassana meditation retreat instead. It was the hardest thing I've ever done, like climbing El Capitan. Every day I wanted to bail, the pain was so distracting at first. When I would bring my attention to my thumb, the sensations were so intense. But as I moved my attention around, the pain lessened; it was really amazing to see how my attention affected my experience of pain.

THE TAKEAWAY

This might seem like a lot of complex information, but this is your body! It is complex, capable, resilient, and amazing. Learning more about how your body works and how to support your overall health will help you enjoy the trail life for many decades to come. Take time to get familiar with your anatomy and let it deepen your body awareness on and off the trail. The biggest points to take away are:

- Take time to prepare your whole body and mind for the trail by practicing daily.

- Yoga can help improve overall balance, strength, endurance, and body awareness, which can better prepare you for the trail.

- While a lot of focus may be on the legs and lower body, don't neglect your core and upper body in your preparation for backpacking and hiking.

- A well-rounded practice will support the back body, which often is underused and even sleepy, while helping open up the front body, which tends to be chronically tight. As you can see from the lists of helpful postures there is a lot of overlap, and a regular, moderate practice will improve your alignment, minimize imbalances, and increase your overall body awareness.

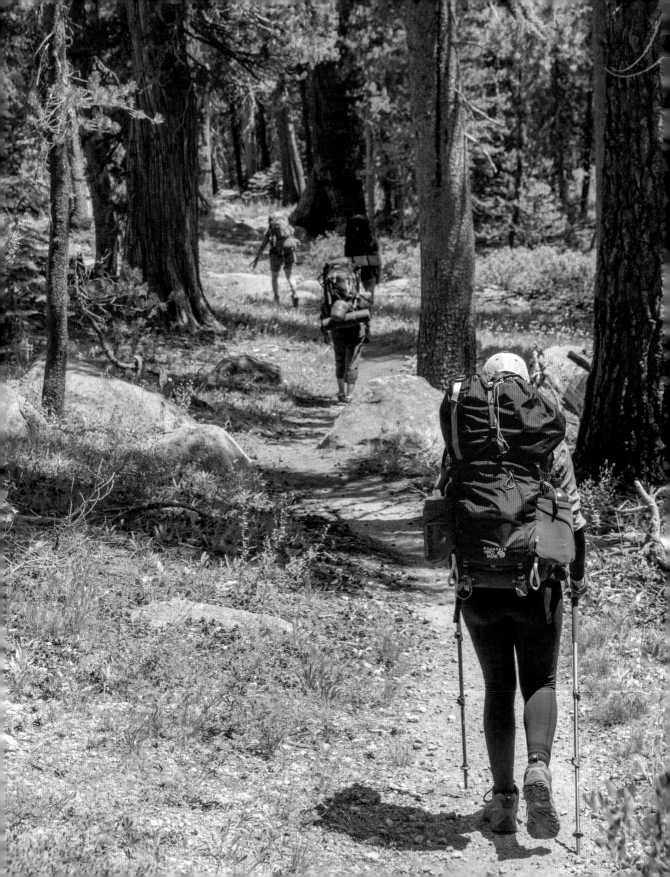

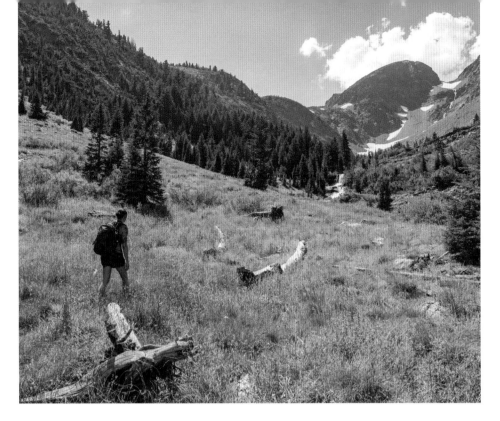

CHAPTER 7

YOGA FOR BACKPACKING

Keep close to Nature's heart . . . and break clear away,
once in awhile, and climb a mountain or spend a
week in the woods. Wash your spirit clean.

—JOHN MUIR

BACKPACKING IS ONE OF MY GREATEST JOYS. It's challenging, breathtaking, and healing. While I had some experience hiking, my first big backpacking trip was in the Annapurna range in central Nepal in my early twenties. My big external-frame pack was stuffed with all the clothes I had to keep me warm in the cold mountain air. I had no idea what I was in for. The first day was incredibly beautiful, and nearly every joint in my body hurt by sunset. As we continued on, though,

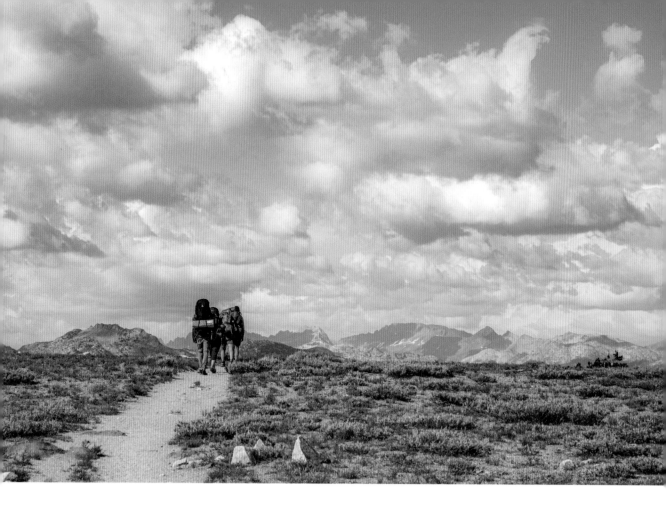

" THOROUGHLY TRAINING FOR BACKPACKING HELPS PREPARE YOU AND ALLOWS YOU TIME TO ADDRESS POSTURAL AND MUSCULAR IMBALANCES TO CREATE MORE MOBILITY AND STRENGTH. PREPARATION INCREASES THE OVERALL ENJOYMENT AND SAFETY OF LONG-DISTANCE HIKING."

winding through rhododendron forests, past waterfalls and moss-covered boulders, all my senses were alive. I felt I was gliding over the trail with ease, barely aware of my pack. The next couple of days were spent reveling in the views, the kindness of my companions, and the bliss of yak butter tea and fried bread from the teahouses. I was in heaven. However, after our descent I was stiff and aching. Thankfully a friend showed me some yoga postures and I found profound relief. It was as if I had been handed two golden tickets: backpacking and yoga.

Something profound and magical happens when I get out into the mountains and reach a stunning vista, which makes all the physical challenge worth it. There is an itch I get when I have been at sea level too long. I yearn to get a higher vantage of the world around me. It helps me make sense of things to get above the minutiae of life and see the simple beauty of nature. Practicing yoga helps me get out on the trails and go farther with greater body/mind awareness. It helps me be more deeply connected to my surroundings. It also helps me address physical imbalances, improve my breath capacity, and recover from backpacking.

ANATOMY OF BACKPACKING

Backpacking takes us deeper into the wilderness than day hiking can. Terrain and altitude vary greatly on longer treks. Carrying your gear, hiking long distances, and being at higher elevations challenges every part of us. Physically we are carrying more weight for longer periods, putting more pressure on the body. If we are heading to higher elevations, the lungs will be challenged even more to get the oxygen needed to keep going and stay clear-headed. Training is necessary.

The demands on the body are similar to hiking yet with the added weight of a full pack. It requires strong legs, core, back, and shoulders as well as greater breath capacity and endurance. Depending on the length of the trip, a pack can weigh anywhere from 25 to 60 pounds. This puts more pressure on the shoulders, spine, and lower body. Adding weight challenges our posture, causing any imbalances to reveal themselves. Hike as much as you can before a trip, slowly adding more weight to a pack as you get closer to your backpacking trip. Thoroughly training for backpacking helps prepare you and allows you time to address postural and muscular imbalances to create more mobility and strength. Preparation increases the overall enjoyment and safety of long-distance hiking.

Feet

As we move along changing terrain, our feet move through dorsiflexion (flexed), plantar flexion (pointed), eversion (sole of foot facing outward), and inversion (sole of foot facing inward). Having shoes that are wide in the toe box with good arch support allows the toes to spread and the arches to disperse weight through the foot. The ankles will be challenged as we navigate trails with extra weight. Try to walk through the length of your foot from heel to toes. Push down through the foot to move forward instead of lifting from the hip flexors. As we push through the foot, the calf muscles—gastrocnemius and soleus—will engage as well as the anterior tibialis on the front of the shin and peroneal muscles on the outer shin. Keeping the feet, ankles, and lower legs strong and flexible will also help minimize ankle injuries. Create flexibility and strength by using tennis balls to massage your feet, walking

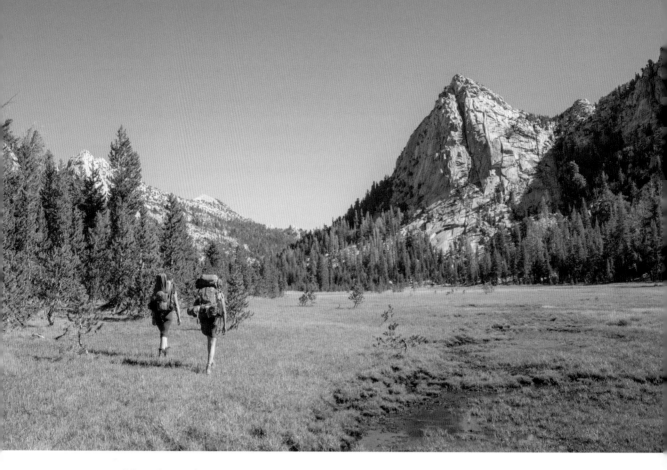

around barefoot when you can, and practicing yoga. Postures that are helpful are downward facing dog, child's pose, toe stretching pose, and standing postures such as side angle pose and the warrior poses.

Legs

The legs should carry most of the load as you backpack. Walking through the length of your feet and pushing down to move forward engages the lower leg muscles and helps engage the muscles of the thigh more evenly. As we walk, the quadriceps and inner thigh muscles engage to straighten the leg, the glutes engage to help extend the hip, and the hamstrings engage to flex the knee. If your quadriceps and hip flexors tend to be tighter from lots of sitting, the hamstrings and hip muscles will not engage properly. Try to drive your weight down through your feet and feel your hamstrings and gluteal muscles engage as you hike. Carrying a pack tends to force the upper body to lean forward slightly, which tightens the hip flexors. Pushing off through your feet and engaging the back of the legs counterbalances this.

When hiking uphill, keep your core engaged as you lift your leg and keep your standing leg firmly grounded. The psoas and quadriceps femoris engage to lift the leg, and keeping the navel drawn in and up helps stabilize the low back and increase balance. As we hike, the inner thigh muscles also engage to aid in balance and stability of the knee. Balancing postures such as tree pose, dancer pose, half moon, and warrior three are excellent for strengthening the hamstrings and quadriceps. Postures such as hand to big toe pose, triangle, wide legged forward fold, standing forward fold, and seated forward fold all help lengthen the hamstrings and strengthen the quadriceps. Lunges, warrior one and two, and all backbends are helpful for strengthening the hamstrings. Working with a varied practice brings greater balance to the muscles of the legs and can decrease muscle fatigue and knee strain.

Hips/Low Back

The hips (our center of gravity) carry the bulk of pack weight. On the front of the pelvis, the hip flexors, including the iliopsoas, engage as we walk and lean slightly forward. This slight lean forward to accommodate extra weight puts more strain on the psoas muscle and the low back. As the gluteus maximus and minimus engage, the leg goes into extension supported by the hamstrings. With each step gluteus medius and tensor fascia latae engage along with the lateral rotators to stabilize the pelvis. The hips are constantly working as we hike, and muscle imbalances can cause strain on the knees below and the low back above. Pay special attention to stretching and strengthening the hips through a varied yoga practice. Postures that are especially helpful are forward fold in easy pose, pigeon pose, fire log pose, head to knee pose, dancer pose, and hero pose.

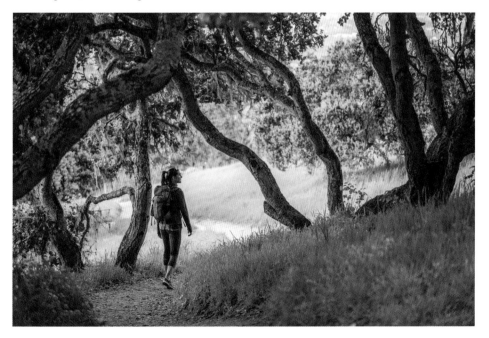

Torso/Core

Good alignment and engagement of the trunk of the body helps keep the low back and spine healthy and aids in even distribution of weight. Remember that the core of your body runs from your pelvis to the shoulders and centers around the spine. A strong core, back, and shoulders will help you carry the weight of your pack longer and with less fatigue and injury. It is common for beginning backpackers to flex the spine too much, creating a hunched position of the spine and shoulders. Try to lift up through your abdominal muscles and feel your back muscles, the erectors along the spine, and the rhomboids between the shoulders engage. Let the trapezius muscles on the tops of your shoulders relax. Let your pelvis, legs, and core carry the weight instead of your shoulders. Engaging through the abdominals and upper back will also take the strain off the low back by keeping the spine supported and long.

Strengthen all sides of the core to prepare for backpacking. Hold plank pose and side plank pose for 30 to 60 seconds three to five times during your practice three times a week. Plank engages all the core muscles, especially the rectus abdominis and the transverse abdominis, which help to stabilize the spine and low back. Side plank engages the internal and external obliques on the sides of the torso. Boat pose, half boat pose, and bicycles are all excellent practices to strengthen all the abdominal muscles, as are all standing balancing postures. Backbends such as locust, cobra, upward facing dog, and full wheel help strengthen the back muscles and shoulders to support posture.

Shoulders/Arms/Neck

While hiking, the shoulders are fairly relaxed with slight engagement of the rhomboids between the shoulder blades. This slight engagement of the rhomboids also helps align the neck, reducing strain. The cervical spine has a natural curve, but a forward head position is very common these days due to overuse of devices. Try to keep your eyes ahead on the trail or horizon to keep from looking down at your feet and straining your neck. With the spine and shoulders in good alignment, the arms will swing naturally. This helps with balance and creates a gentle twisting motion through the torso. Using hiking poles will engage the arms and shoulders, help with overall balance, and reduce swelling in the hands. Lifting and lowering your pack when putting it on and taking it off does require strength in the wrists, forearms, biceps, and triceps. Since there is very little pulling during yoga practice, strengthening the biceps by lifting a weighted pack is helpful for trip preparation. Plank poses and backbends also help with overall shoulder stability and upper back strength. I find headstand and shoulderstand postures incredibly beneficial for upper body alignment, releasing tight shoulder muscles and reducing swelling and fatigue of the lower body after long days on the trail.

SEQUENCES FOR BACKPACKING

Use these sequences to prepare for and recover from your weekly training hikes. Explore the mid-trek postures while you are out when you stop for a rest. Remember to move off the trail to allow others to pass. Many of these postures can be done either lying down on a mat or sitting in a chair to be more accessible.

Pre-trek Sequence

This short practice warms up all the major muscles needed for backpacking. It helps align the spine and strengthen the legs, hips, and core muscles while improving balance.

(1) Upward salute pose
(2) Standing crescent pose
(3) Forward fold
(4) Horse stance with twists
(5) Wide legged forward fold
(6) Warrior one, two, and three
(7) Side angle pose
(8) Hand to big toe pose
(9) Dancer pose
(10) Standing pigeon pose
(11) Downward facing dog pose
(12) Forward fold
(13) Mountain pose

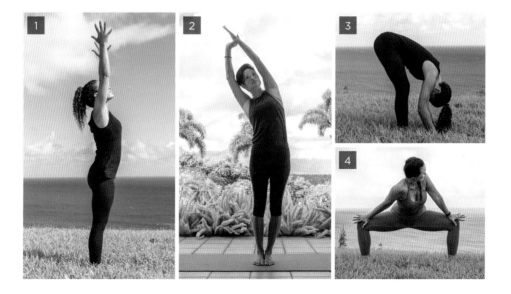

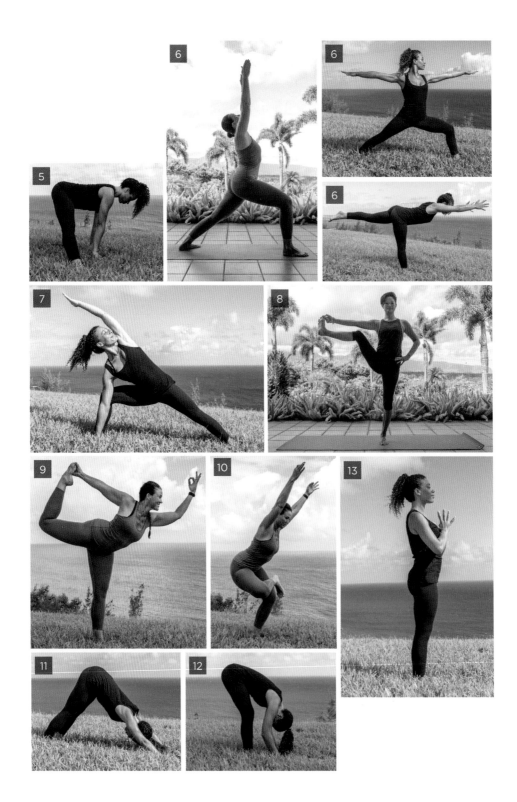

Mid-trek

This sequence is perfect during a longer break in trekking before heading out on the trail again. It helps release muscle tension in the shoulders, hips, legs, and back and prepares the body for the next long stretch of trail.

(1) Upward salute pose
(2) Standing pigeon pose
(3) Forward fold
(4) Triangle pose
(5) Supported backbend pose over a log or boulder
(6) Garland pose
(7) Simple seated twist

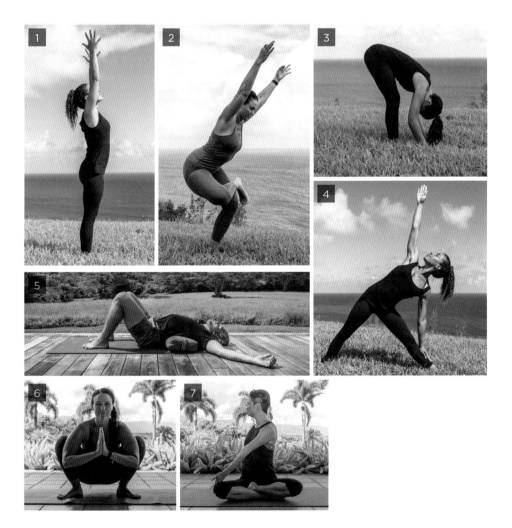

Post-trek Sequence

Try this sequence at the end of your long days of trekking to help unwind the body and release the nervous system's tension. Special attention is given to opening the chest and hips and lengthening the back and leg muscles to help you recover faster.

(1) Sun salutation A (2–6 times) (see page 70)
(2) Dancer pose
(3) Wide legged forward fold with clasped hands
(4) Twisted thigh stretch
(5) Downward facing dog pose
(6) Locust pose
(7) Cobra pose
(8) Lizard lunge
(9) Upward facing dog pose
(10) Bow pose
(11) One-legged royal pigeon pose
(12) Bridge pose or full wheel pose
(13) Head to knee pose
(14) Seated wide legged forward fold
(15) Reclined twist
(16) Happy baby pose
(17) Shoulderstand or candlestick pose
(18) Headstand variation
(19) Corpse pose (stay for at least 5 minutes)
(20) *Nadi shodhana* (10 rounds)
(21) Meditation

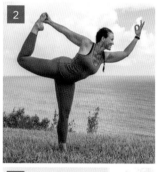
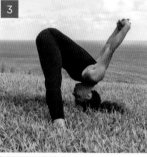
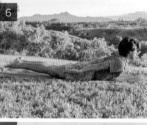
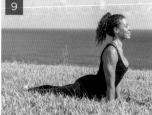
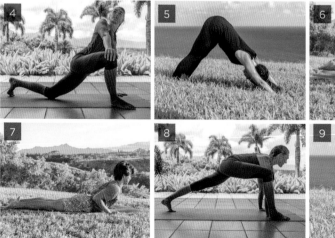

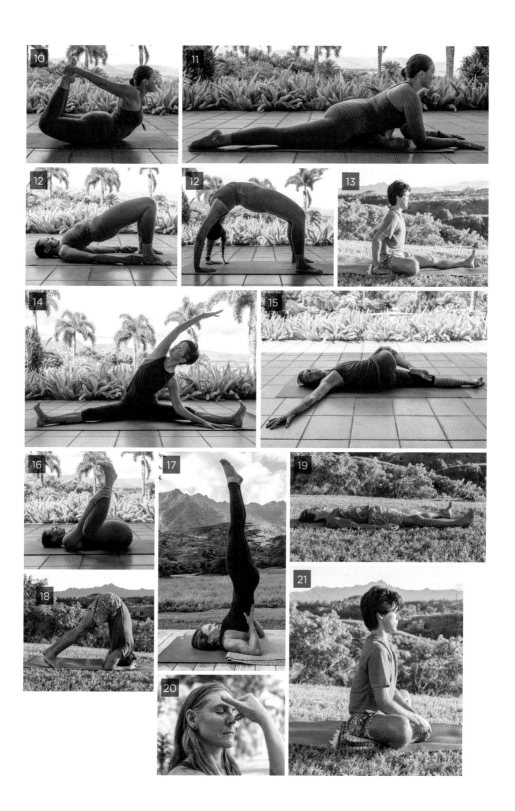

THE TAKEAWAY

Backpacking has all the demands of hiking yet with the added challenge of pack weight. Hiking as much as you can to train for a backpacking trip helps immensely in your overall fitness and preparation. However, adding some targeted strength training and yoga practice helps even more. Backpacking at elevation over varied terrain in the wilderness demands greater mind-body awareness, cardiovascular health, and strength.

- Added weight from a pack forces the body to lean forward at the hips and can challenge the low back and shoulders.

- Increased weight also reveals any imbalances in the body; the ankles, knees, and low back are especially vulnerable.

- Practicing more standing poses, balancing postures, and core work helps prepare the body for backpacking.

- Hip openers, forward bends, and backbends are all necessary to counterbalance long days of hiking with a pack.

- Meditation and breathwork help increase mental awareness and manage stress in the wilderness.

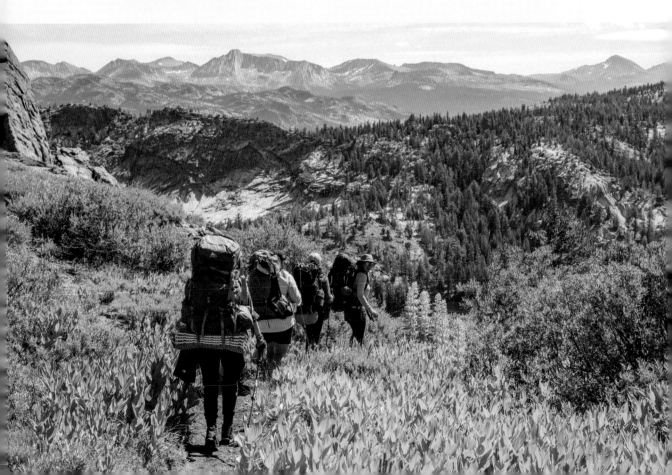

YOGI INSIGHT

DR. BREEZY JACKSON
biologist UC Merced, yoga instructor, and multi-sport athlete; Wawona, CA.

How did you find yoga?
In college I was a Division 1 rower, and my coach had us take a yoga class once per week to help build mental acuity and improve our performance. Beyond the mental benefits yoga really helped me become more physically centered, which is key for rowing. It also helped me see muscular imbalances from a different perspective. Instead of focusing on more core strength to help my pelvic alignment, I realized I needed to release my tight hip flexors.

Does your yoga practice change depending on the sport you are engaging in daily?
Not really. I have a daily practice that focuses on addressing my personal needs to create balanced mobility and strength. It prepares me for any activity I do. My practices after backpacking are more specific, focusing on the external rotators of the hips, the hip flexors, and the chest.

How has your yoga practice influenced your backpacking and other sports?
In general my yoga practice has shifted my mindset from being competitive to being focused on the experience. I want to be as engaged and aware as possible physically, mentally, and spiritually, whether I am backpacking, climbing, cycling, or anything else.

Do you think your yoga practice has helped you with injuries?
Definitely. It helps me recover faster from an injury and also prevent injury by managing risks and helping me check my ego.

What do you love about backpacking specifically?
The accessibility. It's one of the few ways to get into remote locations in the backcountry and experience the beauty of nature. I also really value the self-reliance of carrying what I need on my back, making do with what I have, and the simplicity of living it creates. In the modern world we have access to so much, but in the backcountry, if you didn't bring it with you, you learn to use what you have. There is a certain level of non-attachment that's healthy.

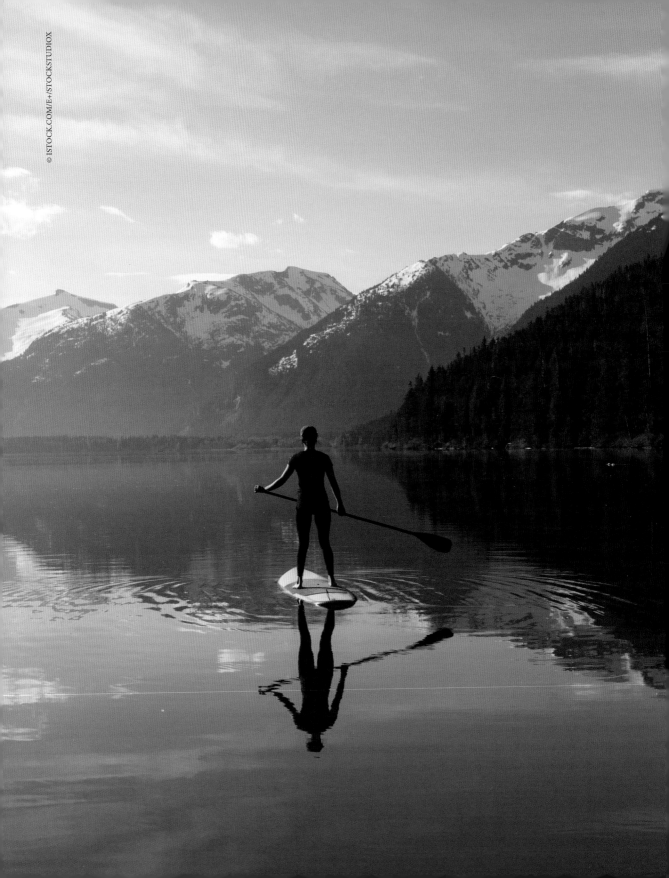

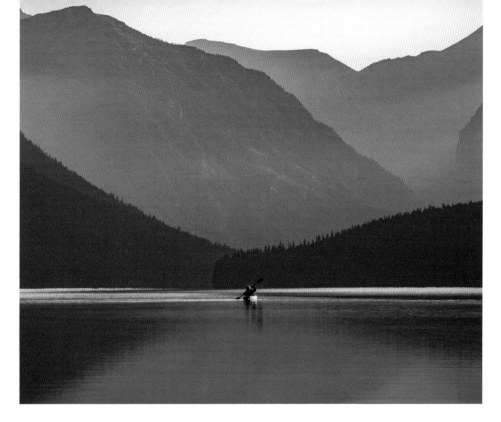

CHAPTER 8

YOGA FOR PADDLING

There are many ways to salvation, and one of them is to follow a river.
—DAVID BROWER

GLIDING ALONG THE RIVER NEAR MY CHILDHOOD HOME in Florida, peeking into the depths to spy on the fish, turtles, manatees, and dolphins while herons and pelicans hunted for their meals was absolute bliss. Later, learning to navigate the currents and exploring bigger rivers in Pennsylvania and Michigan tested my skills and brought me to places with profound beauty and serenity. Moments connected to the currents, basking in the sun, watching birds and dragonflies brought all my senses alive and that deep peace that is described in the *Yoga Sutras* as *santosha*, contentment.

Ancient yoga texts claim that bliss and peace are our natural state—we just need to set up the right conditions to experience it. For some, the right conditions are a vessel, a paddle, and a long stretch of water. Time in nature is a gateway to this bliss

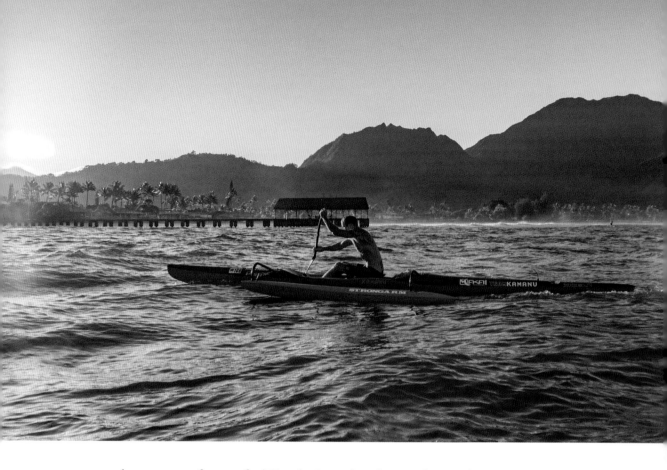

state that any one of us can find. You don't need to fly to India, stand on your head, or spend hours chanting. You just need to get outside. There is a peace and grace in nature that has always captivated and drawn me into its secrets. It's where I feel most myself, most alive, most in tune. It is endlessly fascinating to explore, and thankfully humans have created myriad tools to access its beauty.

Since moving to Hawaii I've begun to explore the rivers and streams on paddleboards and am learning the art of outrigger canoeing. While the surf might be full of locals and visitors, there is a large and active community of paddlers exploring the rivers and streams as well. No matter what your drive is for paddling, we all face similar physical and mental challenges—balanced strength, breath control, and focus. We can all benefit from a regular yoga practice that helps us to both counter and support the rigors of paddling life.

Paddling demands strength and endurance of the legs, core, and shoulders simultaneously. Unlike hiking and cycling, which are very lower body dominant, paddling demands the whole body be in balance. The legs and shoulders tend to take over as we get tired, putting the low back and neck at risk for misalignment and injury.

" ANCIENT YOGA TEXTS CLAIM THAT BLISS AND PEACE
ARE OUR NATURAL STATE—WE JUST NEED TO SET UP THE
RIGHT CONDITIONS TO EXPERIENCE IT. FOR SOME, THE RIGHT
CONDITIONS ARE A VESSEL, A PADDLE, AND A LONG STRETCH
OF WATER."

Overall, balance and awareness can help minimize repetitive stress from paddling. Better alignment and holistic muscle recruitment also helps sustain our energy, alertness, and overall connection to nature. This gives us a greater chance of enjoying the ride, faster recovery, and the freedom to get out again a little sooner.

Working to address imbalances and build muscle coordination is crucial for longevity in any sport. It also improves our health and vitality as well as the overall functioning of every system of the body. Good posture improves the functioning of the respiratory, circulatory, and digestive systems. When we hunch over in the shoulders and low back, our lung capacity is greatly reduced and the back of the body gets chronically weakened. This can lead to tight pectorals, diaphragm restriction, and tightness in the hip flexors. Practice postures that open up the front body and strengthen the back to improve posture, endurance, and overall pleasure of paddling.

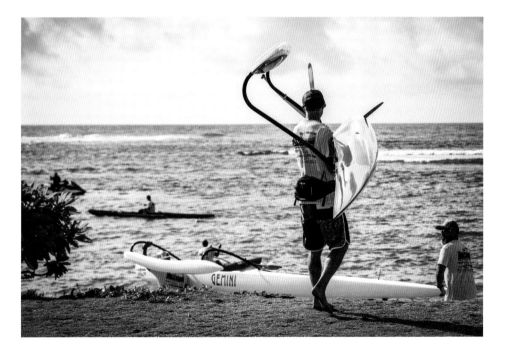

ANATOMY OF PADDLING

While paddling in a kayak or canoe, or on a paddleboard, the lower body is engaged in isometric contraction, creating stability that requires enduring strength. The lower body joints are fixed into position, and there is a rooting downward from the pelvis to the feet. Let's take a deeper look at the lower body muscles and their involvement in paddling.

Feet

Depending on what you are paddling, the feet are either in dorsiflexion, meaning the ankle is flexed and the heel is rooting downward, or in plantar flexion (foot is pointed) and pressing through the balls of the feet. In dorsiflexion, the shin muscles are shortened, which can put strain on the patellar ligament and the knee. In plantar flexion the calf muscles—gastrocnemius and soleus—are chronically contracted, placing strain on the Achilles tendon and plantar fascia of the feet. Keeping the feet active during paddling helps support the natural curves of the spine. Pressing evenly through the feet helps with balance and integration of the legs and core.

Our feet are shaped by our history, shoes, and activity or lack thereof, leading most everyone to have imbalances in the feet that are carried up the body. It really all starts here. So take some time to work with your feet. Create flexibility and strength by using tennis balls to massage your feet, walking around barefoot when you can, and practicing yoga.

Legs

While kayaking or canoeing, the feet, knees, and hips are in a flexed position for long periods of time. The muscles of the thighs are typically in a lengthened yet contracted state, while the muscles in the back of the legs (calves and hamstrings) are in a shortened and contracted state. The quadriceps are heavily engaged in bracing the legs during paddling, and the iliacus and psoas work to flex the hip and trunk. This tension in the quads and hip flexors, coupled with tight hamstrings, often causes tension and misalignment in the low back and pelvis as well as greater torque on the knees. Try to engage the backs of the legs, hamstrings, and glutes while paddling by pulling back through the heels to take the load off the quadriceps muscles.

Hips/Low Back

Since there are so many attachment sites for muscles on all sides of the pelvis, imbalances can cause chronic tension patterns that relay up the spine and affect posture. The quadriceps, hip flexors, tensor fascia latae, and deep adductors all attach to the front of the pelvis. These stabilizing muscles are constantly used in balancing and can cause strain on the knees. On the back of the pelvis is the gluteus maximus,

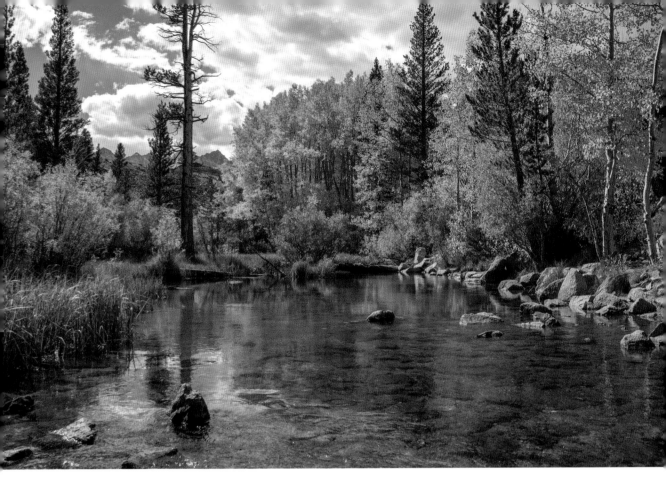

which extends and internally rotates the hip. Six deep lateral rotators attach to the back of the pelvis beneath the gluteus maximus. These deeper muscles tend to be weaker and tighter, as they're easily overpowered by the gluteus maximus. One in particular, the piriformis, can impinge the sciatic nerve that runs through the pelvis, causing sciatica. The gluteus medius lies on the lateral side of the hip to stabilize but is often underused and sleepy. Practicing standing postures, backbends, and hip opening postures can help correct deep imbalances and improve the health of the pelvis and posture.

Torso/Core

Good alignment allows the entire trunk of the body to engage while paddling, distributing the work and weight more evenly. Sit on the flat of your sit bones with your feet planted. Draw your low belly in and upward, and the shoulders back slightly and down away from your ears. Lengthen the back of your neck and extend upward through your crown as much as you can as you paddle. Most paddlers are seated, so the hips are flexed. The torso tends to flex as well if the backline isn't

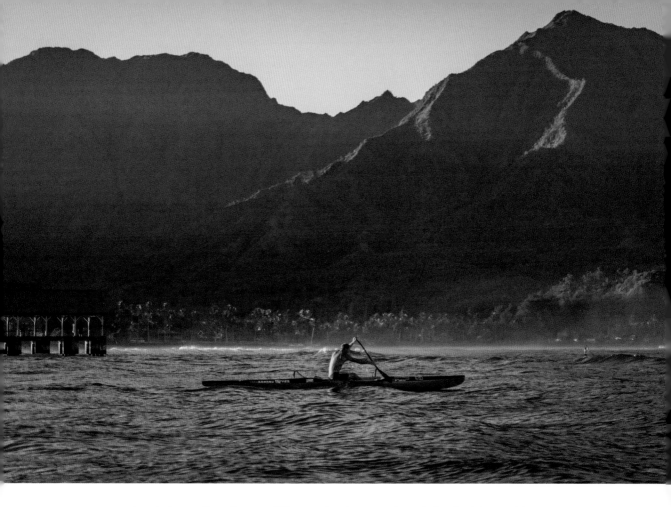

engaged to balance. Stand-up paddlers maintain more length in the hips and lower torso, and the trunk flexes with each stroke.

The chest muscles (pectoralis major and minor) are constantly in demand during paddling of any sort and need lengthening. All four layers of abdominal muscles are also engaged throughout paddling, with the superficial rectus abdominis being dominant. Engaging the obliques facilitates rotation and side flexion of the trunk, taking pressure off the shoulders and arms as well as driving power down through the legs.

On the back of the trunk, the serratus anterior draws the shoulder forward to paddle and is often very tight. The latissimus dorsi runs from the shoulders down the back in a diamond shape connecting to the spine. It is a powerful muscle that is responsible for shoulder adduction, extension, and internal rotation as well as extension and lateral flexion of the lower lumbar spine. It plays a vital role in shoulder and low back health. Just below the lattisimus dorsi is the quadratus lumborum, which laterally flexes the trunk and also extends the lumbar. It plays a role in low back health and sacroiliac stability as well.

Shoulders/Neck/Arms

The shoulder is another ball-and-socket joint, but shallower and less stable than the hip. Numerous muscles work together to create stability and mobility here where the humerus meets the scapula. On the back are the rhomboid muscles, which run between the upper thoracic spine and the shoulder blades, drawing them toward the midline and also moving them up and down. Smaller muscles surrounding the shoulder blades such as the supraspinatus, subscapularis, infraspinatus, and teres major work together to create the shoulder and upper arm movements, although the posterior muscles (back body) are often underused, leading to rotator cuff injuries for paddlers.

Levator scapulae, splenius, sternocleidomastoid (SCM), and scalenes are the primary neck muscles. Paddlers tend to flex the neck forward, shearing the cervical vertebrae and creating more pressure on the discs, especially with rotation of the neck. The SCM and scalenes get tight pulling the head forward, causing the levator and splenius to shorten and tighten as well. Working to stabilize the posterior shoulders and create more mobility in the shoulder joints helps reduce pressure and misalignment on the neck.

While the torso and legs are fully engaged during paddling, the arms tend to do most of the work—especially for beginners. Engaging through the core and using

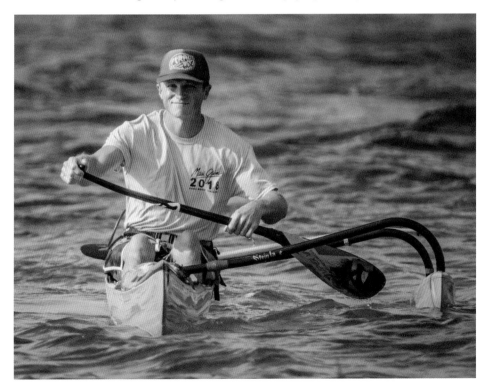

the legs comes with time and practice. The biceps brachii flexes the shoulder and elbow and supinates the forearm (rotates to palm upward position). The triceps brachii extends both the shoulder and the elbow during the sweeping-back motion of paddling. Smaller muscles control the forearms and wrists. The gripping muscles tend to be very tight, while the top of the forearm and wrist tend to be weak. This can lead to both elbow and wrist issues for paddlers.

SEQUENCES FOR PADDLING

Many of these postures can be done either lying down on a mat or sitting in a chair to be more accessible.

Pre-paddle Sequence

This sequence is for warming up all the major muscles before setting out on the water.

(1) Joint rotations (see pages 49–51)
(2) Horse stance with twists
(3) Sun salutations: classical with low lunge (3–6 times) (see page 70)
(4) Wide legged forward fold with clasped hands
(5) Low lunge pose
(6) Dancer pose
(7) Simple seated twist
(8) Seated forward fold

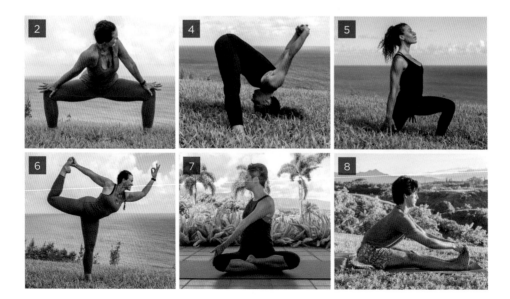

Mid-paddle

Pause at some point in your paddling to stretch the neck, shoulders, arms, and back to ease any strain and reignite your energy. You can do these postures and movements sitting in your kayak or on the shore. Hold the paddle with your hands about 3 to 4 feet apart and push up against the paddle to engage the shoulder muscles as you perform the poses.

(1) Upward salute pose (with paddle)
(2) Side stretch (with paddle)
(3) Neck rolls
(4) Wrist rolls
(5) Seated cat/cow poses
(6) Seated forward fold
(7) Simple seated twist

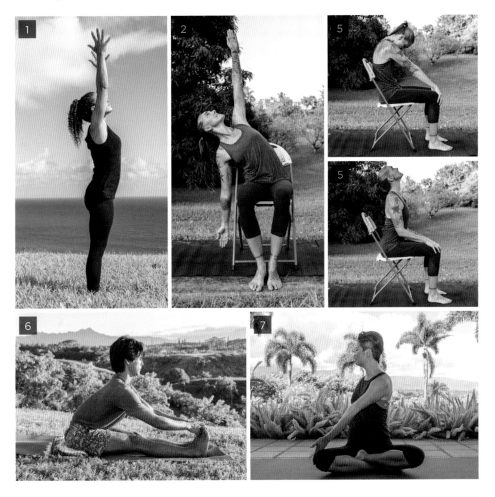

Post-paddle Sequence

This sequence should be done on shore after you are done paddling for the day. It helps bring mobility and suppleness to all the muscles and joints and improves recovery.

(1) Mountain pose
(2) Forward fold
(3) Low lunge pose
(4) Runner's stretch
(5) Downward facing dog pose
(6) Cobra or upward facing dog pose
(7) Warrior two pose
(8) Side angle pose
(9) Triangle pose
(10) Half moon pose
(11) Wide legged forward fold
(12) Tree pose
(13) Dancer pose
(14) Standing pigeon pose
(15) Dolphin pose
(16) Cow faced pose
(17) Bridge/wheel pose
(18) Reclined twist
(19) Happy baby pose
(20) Reclined knees to chest pose
(21) Child's pose
(22) Head to knee pose
(23) Simple seated twist
(24) Windshield wiper pose
(25) Reclined hand to big toe pose variations
(26) Corpse pose
(27) Meditation

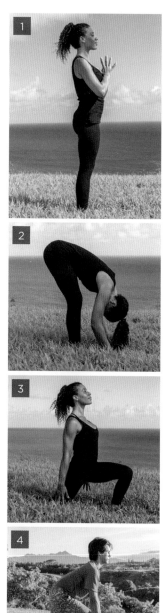

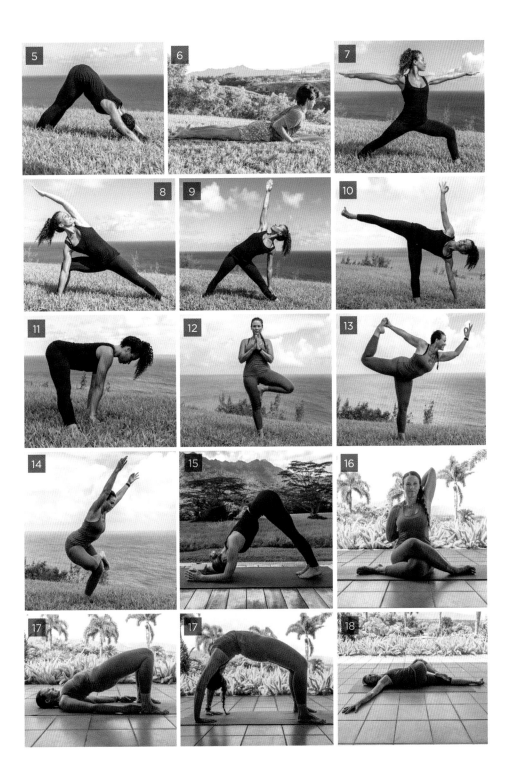

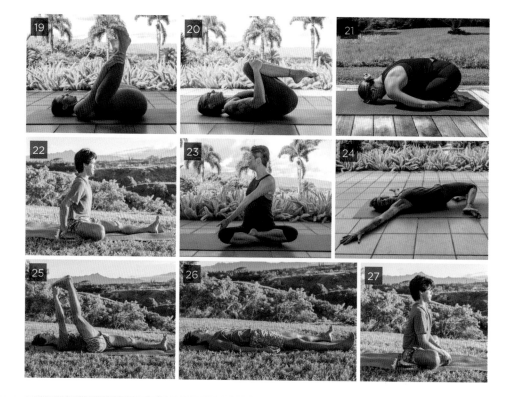

THE TAKEAWAY

Whether you are a water-sport newbie or a longtime paddler, incorporating a yoga practice into your routine can greatly enhance your time on the water. By increasing body awareness, improving balance and alignment, and expanding breath capacity, each stroke becomes more graceful.

- Take the time to prepare the body, mind, and soul for a paddle.

- While paddling maintain a strong foundation through your feet, legs, and hips by rooting.

- Maintain a lift through the core and stabilize the shoulders while paddling.

- Pause for stretching overhead and to the sides and back sometime during your paddle.

- A short practice after a paddle gives us time to pause, thank the environment and our bodies, and integrate that paddle experience deeper into our lives.

YOGI INSIGHT

ANNA LEVESQUE

professional kayaker, yoga teacher and Ayurvedic
practitioner, founder Mind Body Paddle; NC.

How did you get into kayaking?
When I was nineteen I took a job at a summer rafting camp working in the
kitchen. At the time I was going to school for law, but once I found paddling and
kayaking I was hooked. Kayaking taught me how to live well. You have no choice
but to be in the present moment.

How does having a yoga practice help support your paddling?
It's absolutely a necessity. If I didn't have my daily yoga practice I don't know
if I would still be paddling. It reduces injury, increases my body awareness, and
keeps me healthy, mobile, and enjoying life.

What do you love about paddling and yoga?
Paddling teaches me presence and courage. Yoga is part of my Ayurvedic
lifestyle and really helps with recovery, increasing my breath awareness, and
improving my alignment. Yoga is a discipline that reduces pain and keeps me
healthy and paddling.

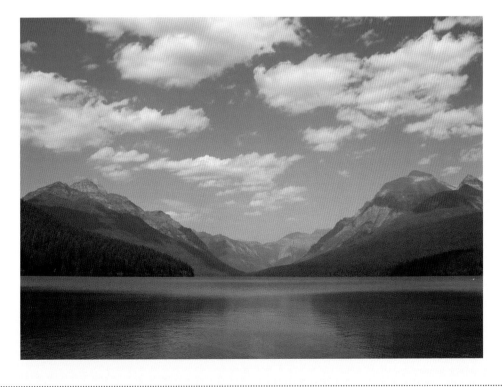

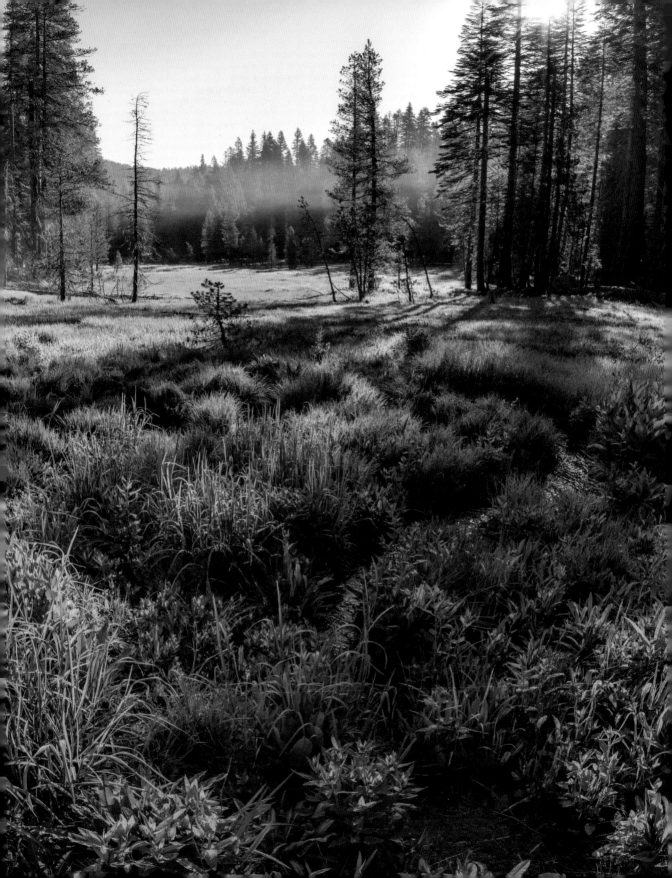

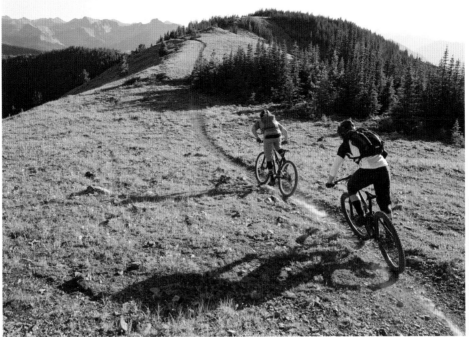

CHAPTER **9**

YOGA FOR CYCLING

When the spirits are low, when the day appears dark, when
work becomes monotonous, when hope hardly seems worth
having, just mount a bicycle and go out for a spin down the road,
without thought on anything but the ride you are taking.

—ARTHUR CONAN DOYLE

LEARNING TO RIDE A BIKE was one of the most thrilling days of my life. I was so
eager to be free of my training wheels and tear off down the street on my own. My
father followed me around the driveway and street for hours the first time I was free
of the training wheels. I was so determined to do it on my own that when I finally
got my speed and balance to click, I took off down the road, my dad chasing after
me and cheering me on. That feeling of absolute freedom and bliss was addictive,
and I was on my bike streaking off into the distance every chance I got after that.

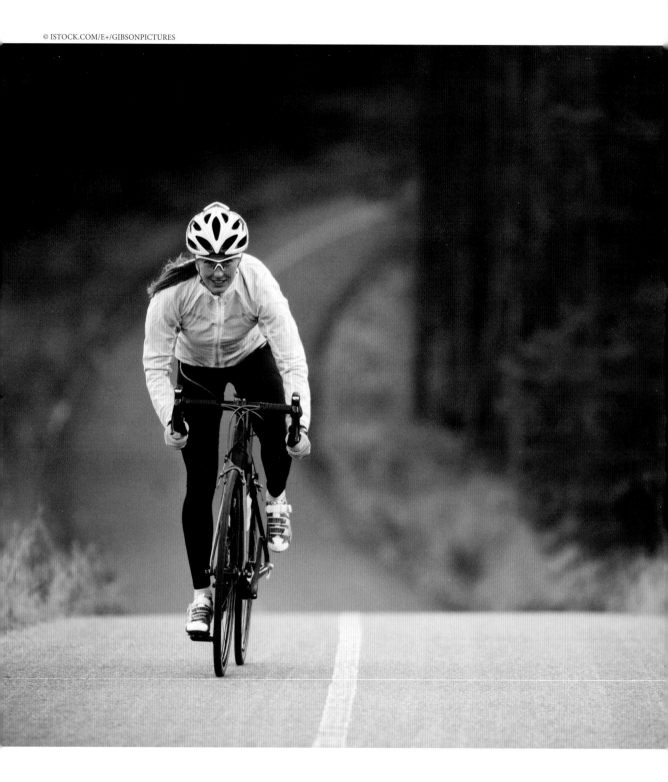

Years later, in my early twenties, my bike became my main mode of transportation. As soon as spring thawed the snow and ice off the roads, I was out on my bike going to classes, work, or visiting friends. More and more time was spent bike commuting for purpose rather than wandering pleasure. But the joy was still there. Life is different observed at the speed of a bicycle. I notice more than when I am driving and can go farther than when I am walking. Every time I get on a bike I feel like a kid again—exuberant, curious, and somehow untamed.

Riding out in the open or on a trail through the woods engages my entire body, mind, and spirit. There are times when every worry fades away and the peace and beauty of nature overwhelms me. I feel like I could ride forever, flying over the land with ease. Then there are the hills that force me to dig in and find untapped strength and grit to climb higher and see farther. I am always left spent, grateful, and inspired. Cycling can be pure joy. It also can bring pain and suffering. Crashing, long hills, an aching back and shoulders are all part of the cycling life. Yoga not only helps me be more prepared mentally and physically for these demands and challenges, but also helps me along the ride and the recovery afterward.

Cycling is one of the most challenging sports, requiring constant repetition, mental toughness, keen senses, and physical endurance. The demands for energy push the boundaries of our mental and physical capacity. Riding high mileage or on rugged mountain trails requires every part of the body and mind to perform and engage. Cardiovascular health and endurance are key to meet the demands on the road or trail, but so are overall strength and agility. Cycling indoors during winter months benefits both road and trail riders by maintaining and increasing both endurance and cardiovascular fitness. Mountain bikers can benefit from getting out on the road to log some miles, do sprint work, and increase endurance, which translates into greater fitness on the trails.

Obviously the legs need to be strong in cycling, but so do the arms, shoulders, core, and back. It really is a full body sport. Riders are seated for long periods of time, which can lead to rounding the low back and sinking in the chest. A regular yoga practice can help relieve pain and tension in these areas. Crashes are inevitable, and yoga provides an excellent way to recover from both acute and chronic injuries. Let's take a closer look at the needs of cyclists.

YOGI INSIGHT

ROBERT HURST
writer and cyclist; Denver, CO.

You have been cycling a long time, what keeps you riding?
There is so much. I've been riding bikes professionally as a bike messenger and for fun for so long. It's the wide-open spaces, being outside, making me happy, and the peace of mind I get when I'm out there. Part of it is this thought that it is my job as a human to get out, work out, and engage. It's easy to lose that, and we have to get it back in order to feel pain, pleasure, and live fully.

How does yoga help your cycling experience?
It helps me recover from cycling, but meditation and mindfulness help me be more grateful and emotionally grounded.

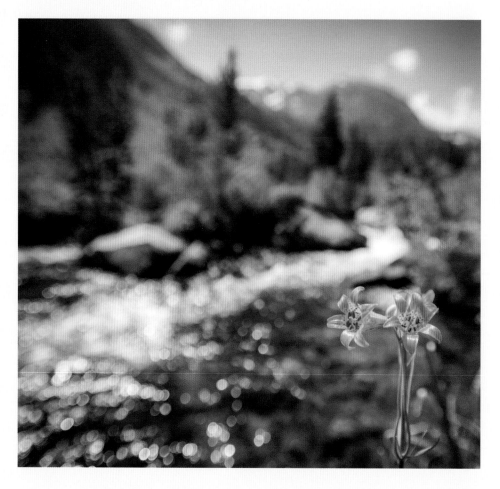

ANATOMY OF CYCLING

Feet/Lower Legs

Cycling is one of those sports where the feet are mostly fixed. The ankles are mainly in dorsiflexion (toes lifting toward knees) while pedaling. Since the feet are bound in shoes, the toes are close together, putting most of the movement into the arches of the feet, ankles, calves, and front of the shin. The ankles are in a predominantly fixed position with subtle movements engaging the calf muscles (soleus and gastrocnemius) and those on the front of the shin (anterior tibialis). Stretching the feet, ankles, and calves is key for recovery and maintaining healthy mobility. Yoga postures that stretch the tops of the feet and front of the shin, like child's pose, seated hero pose, cobra, and locust, are helpful. Postures such as toe stretching pose, downward facing dog pose, cow faced pose, and standing forward fold help stretch calf muscles and the arches of the feet.

Thighs/Knees

While cycling, all the joints of the legs move between 90-degree angles (approximately) to 180-degree angles (neutral or straight), reducing natural range of motion (ROM). The constant seated posture also keeps the hip flexor muscles (psoas and rectus femoris) shorter and often tighter. Hamstrings are equally shortened in the actions of cycling. This leads to concentrated power in the biggest muscles of the legs, but also leads to chronically tight hamstrings and quadriceps for cyclists (the psoas is covered in the hip section). Thankfully yoga has lots of postures that help lengthen both groups of muscles. Some examples of thigh lengthening postures are mountain pose, beginning dancer pose, crescent lunge, low lunge, cobra, warrior one and two poses, bow pose, camel pose, hero pose (seated and reclined), bridge pose, and full wheel pose. As an added benefit many of those postures strengthen the glutes and back as well. Examples of hamstring lengthening postures are standing forward fold, wide legged forward fold, hand to big toe pose, triangle pose, half moon pose, half and full leaping monkey pose, seated forward fold, and plow pose.

Hips/Low Back

Let's face it, sitting for hours is hard on the body, whether it's in front of the computer, TV, or expansive landscape, or on a mountain bike trail. It is especially hard on the low back and hips, increasing compression of the lower spine and intervertebral discs. Although cycling keeps the hips and legs engaged, encouraging the gluteal muscles to stay active, the low back tends to round, especially if the hamstrings are restricted. Bending forward to your handlebars from the pelvis instead of the mid or upper back will help relieve compression of the lower spine. For the most part, road cycling only moves the hips between flexion and neutral, which leads to the hip flexors being chronically short and strong. Navigating mountain bike trails does include lateral movement of the femur/hip joint. The outer hips are typically asleep in most cyclists due to the lack of abduction of the legs, which puts strain on the knees and the pelvis. Postures that lengthen the hamstrings help with low back alignment, and lateral hip postures help to both lengthen and engage the outer hip muscles. Standing pigeon pose, tree pose, warrior two pose, half moon, side plank, fire log pose, and easy sitting pose all engage and lengthen these muscles.

As mentioned above, the hip flexors need some assistance for cyclists. Specifically the iliopsoas and rectus femoris affect the position of the pelvis and low back alignment. Postures that lengthen both the thigh muscles and hip flexors will extend the hip joint and flex the knee joint for maximum benefit. Some postures that meet these goals are dancer pose, twisted thigh stretch, full pigeon (and variations), full wheel pose, half and full frog pose, reclined hero pose, camel pose, and bow pose.

Torso/Core

Cyclists lean forward most of the time, tending to round the spine and collapse the upper body. Focusing on building strength in the abdominal muscles and the back improves posture and endurance and reduces back pain by taking load off the hip flexors and bracing the spine. Leaning forward without lifting the lower belly puts added strain on the low back and tends to keep the breath shallow. Cyclists benefit from yogic breathing and abdominal strengthening to support both their

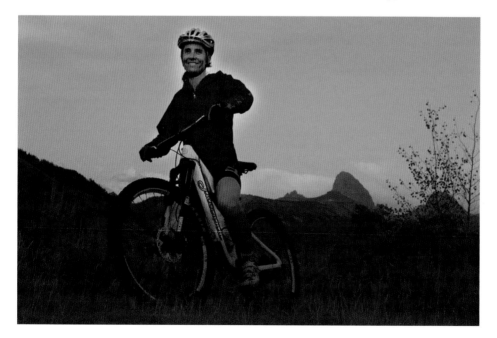

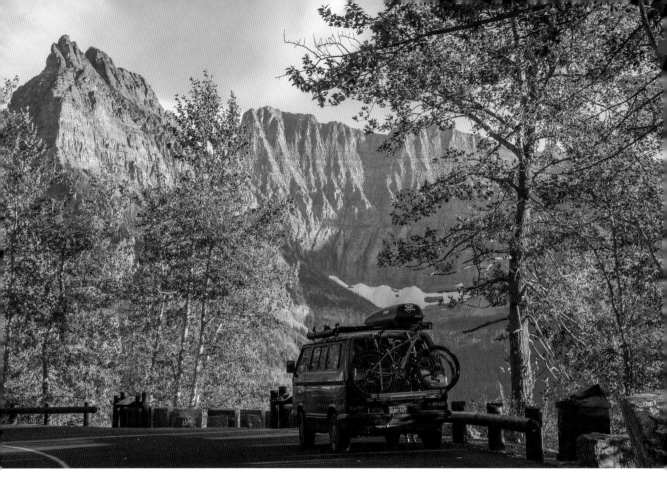

endurance and postural alignment. Strengthening the muscles along the spine and shoulders helps create more length in the torso, improve respiration, and reduce disc compression.

Yoga offers many postures that help lengthen hip flexors and strengthen the back and abdominal muscles. Postures such as warrior one and two, side angle pose, dancer pose, boat pose, cobra pose, locust pose, bow pose, bridge pose, and wheel pose address most of these needs. Plank postures including side plank and four limbed staff pose (*chaturanga dandasana*) help strengthen the core with length in the spine. Standing balancing postures like warrior three and half moon pose and hand balancing postures like crow pose, plank pose, and side plank strengthen the abdominal muscles all around the core. Begin to incorporate some of these postures into every practice.

Upper Body

Holding onto the handlebars for hours means the entire shoulder girdle and arms are constantly engaged. Keeping the grip relaxed whenever possible gives the hands and arms a rest. The shoulders are typically in a protracted position (moving away from spine), which weakens the rhomboids (small stabilizing muscles between the shoulder blades). This positioning also tightens the pectoral muscles in the front of the chest and reduces breathing capacity.

One of the primary goals of the physical side of yoga is to support and strengthen the spine and maximize breathing capacity. Focusing on complete breaths during your yoga practice helps improve upper body posture and increase breath awareness on and off the bike. Postures that extend the spine (backbends) help strengthen muscles on the upper back and along the spine as well as lengthen all the muscles on the front of the chest and the biceps of the upper arms. All postures with the hands on the floor help stretch the hands, wrists, and forearms, while many of the twisting and arm binding postures increase the ROM of the entire arm and shoulder.

SEQUENCES FOR CYCLISTS

Begin practicing the pre-ride and post-ride sequences a few times a week to bring greater balance and mobility to your riding. Use the mid-ride sequences during your training rides when you take a break. If you are competing or doing a longer ride, do a little warming up and focus on the post-ride sequence for recovery. Many of these postures can be done either lying down on a mat or sitting in a chair to be more accessible.

Pre-ride Sequence

Try this sequence regularly before cycling to prepare the major muscles and joints for riding. It also helps wake up all the muscles that support the core and spine for long hours of riding.

(1) Crescent pose
(2) Sun salutation A (5 rounds) (see page 70)
(3) Sun salutation B (5 rounds) (see page 72)
(4) Warrior two pose
(5) Side angle pose
(6) Triangle pose
(7) Wide legged forward fold
(8) Tree pose
(9) Dancer pose
(10) Locust pose
(11) Upward facing dog pose
(12) Downward facing dog pose
(13) Low lunge pose
(14) Standing forward fold
(15) Mountain pose

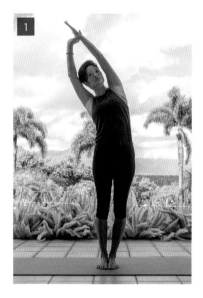

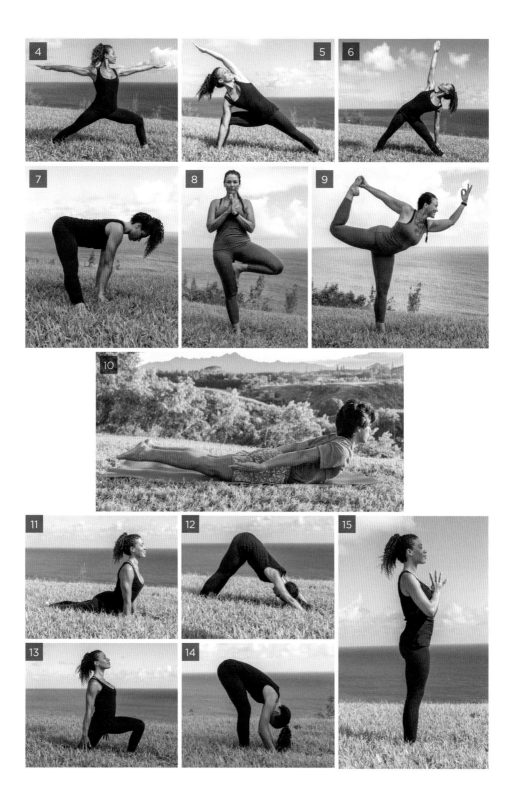

Mid-ride Sequence

On-bike: Do these movements during a short stop on the bike to help relieve muscle tension in the neck, shoulders, and back.

(1) Neck rolls (8 times each direction) (see page 49)

(2) Shoulder rolls (8 times each direction) (see page 49)

(3) Wrist rolls (8 times each direction) (see page 50)

(4) Upward salute pose

(5) Cow faced pose arms

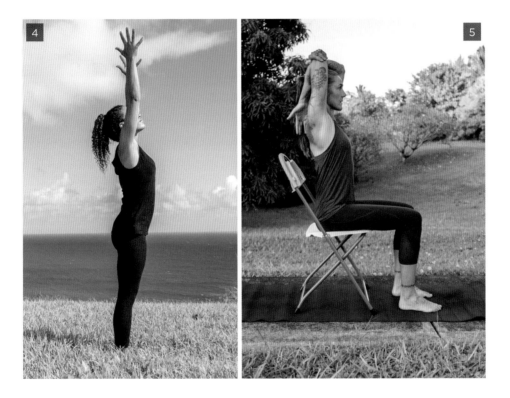

Off-bike: Do these movements during a short break off the bike to address tension in the hips, hamstrings, and back.

(6) Standing forward fold
(7) Crescent lunge
(8) Dancer pose, beginner's variation
(9) Standing pigeon pose
(10) Side angle pose
(11) Wide legged forward fold

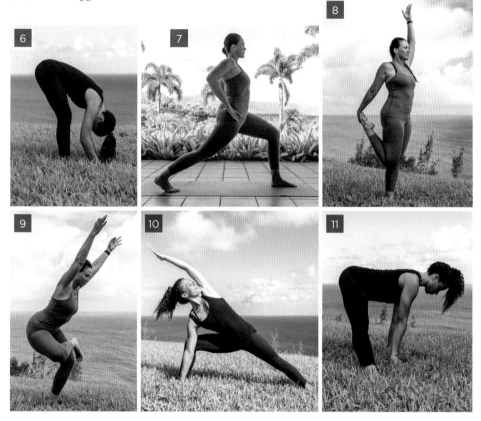

Post-ride Sequence

At the end of a long day of riding, try this sequence to help release muscle tension and fatigue and help the nervous system unwind after the demands of cycling.

(1) Child's pose
(2) Cat/cow poses
(3) Downward facing dog pose
(4) Low lunge pose
(5) Standing forward fold
(6) Spinal rolls
(7) Upward salute pose
(8) Joint rotations
(9) Sun salutation B (2–4 times) (see page 72)
(10) Warrior two pose
(11) Side angle pose
(12) Triangle pose
(13) Half moon pose
(14) Warrior one pose
(15) Downward facing dog pose
(16) Locust pose variations
(17) Cobra rolls
(18) Half frog pose
(19) Downward facing dog pose
(20) Pyramid pose
(21) Revolved triangle pose
(22) Upward facing dog pose
(23) Seated forward fold
(24) Seated wide legged forward fold
(25) Head to knee pose
(26) Simple seated twist
(27) Reclined hero pose, one leg at a time
(28) Bridge pose
(29) Wheel pose
(30) Reclined twist
(31) Happy baby pose
(32) Plow pose
(33) *Nadi shodhana* (5 rounds)
(34) Meditation
(35) Corpse pose

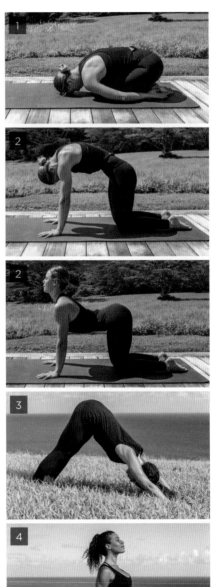

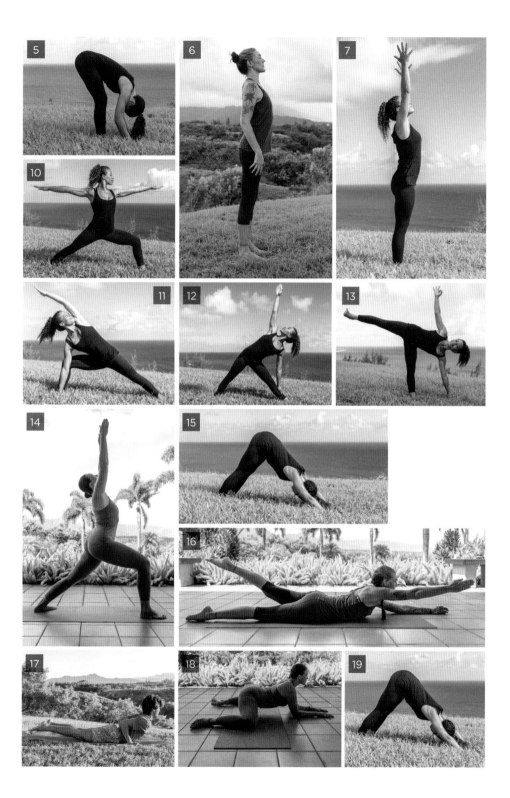

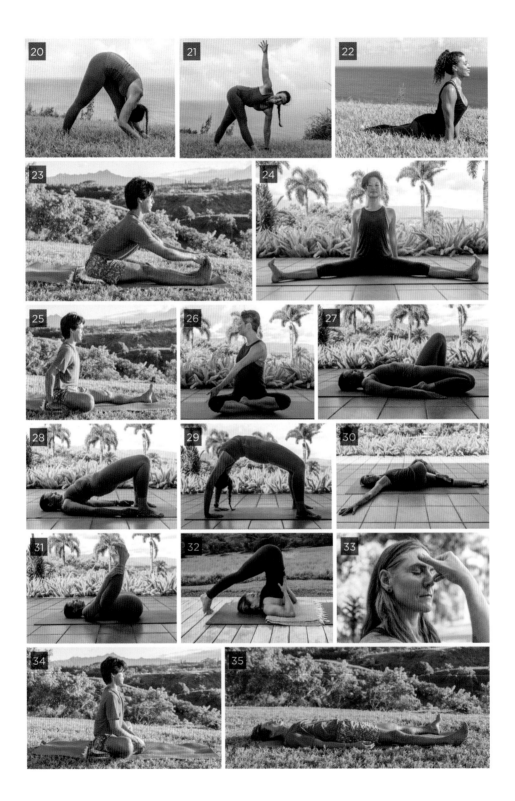

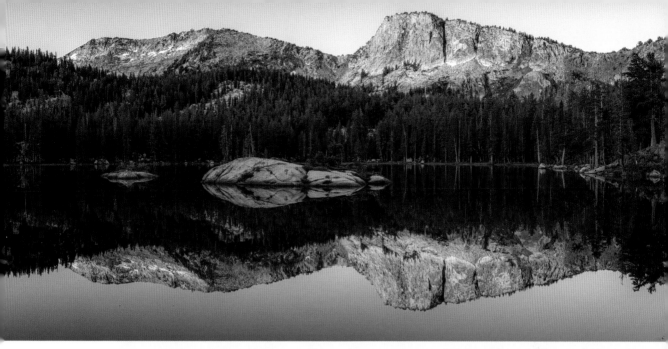

THE TAKEAWAY

Cycling is an incredibly challenging and rewarding outdoor sport. Whether long-distance road cycling or hitting a technical mountain bike trail, the entire body, mind, and spirit are engaged. Flying on two wheels has been exhilarating humans for many years and is one of life's great pleasures. I highly encourage you to dust off your bike, get out on a trail, or hit the open road. Practicing yoga to prepare the body, relieve tension while riding, and speed recovery is an incredible support to the experience. Playing hard has many benefits and challenges. Yoga helps cyclists prepare and face both.

- Cycling requires whole body engagement and fitness. Training the whole body helps increase breath capacity, mental focus, and overall strength.

- Because of the limited movements of the legs and body in cycling, yoga helps cross-train and support whole body fitness.

- Yoga practice helps increase lung capacity and helps the mind stay focused and clear during intense periods of riding.

- Core and upper body strength and mobility help support the spine and especially the low back for cyclists.

- Taking time for a post-ride practice helps cyclists recover faster and enjoy the ride.

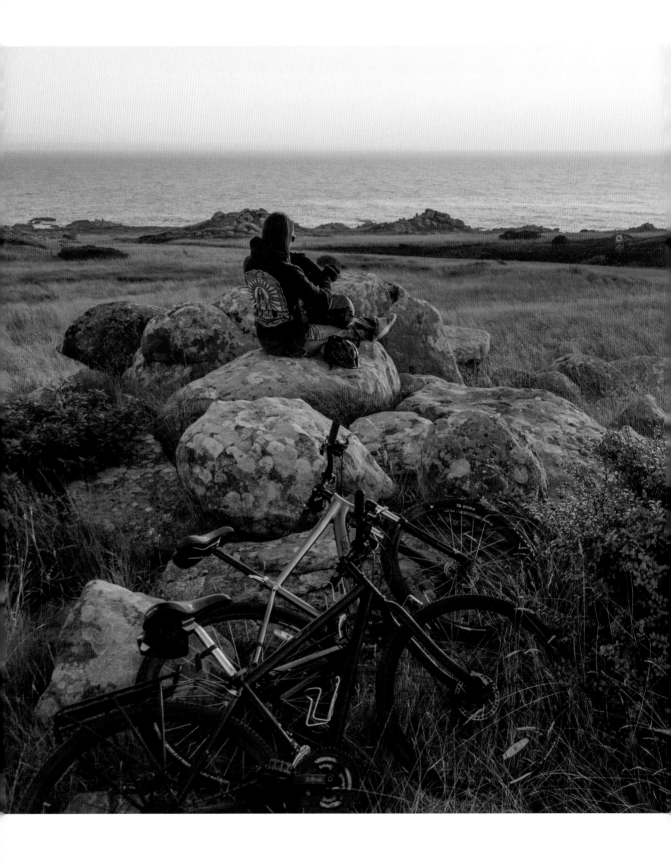

YOGI INSIGHT

GREGG WARNKEN
programmer and artist; Atlanta, GA.

What is it that you love about mountain biking?
I feel like an eight-year-old kid again, playing out in nature, being wild. It brings me back to life and gets me into the flow, totally embodied. The mountain biking community is also really special. It's therapeutic for me. It's also a full body workout and there is nothing like it.

What do you love about being in nature?
I practice shinrin-yoku (forest bathing) while I am out there. I often stop and sit to just soak up nature and get quiet. Being near water also feeds me good energy. Seeing wildlife reminds me I am part of the whole.

How has yoga helped your mountain biking?
I began practicing yoga back in 2002 and have a short morning practice every day. It's made my core much stronger, which increases my agility, stamina, and balance. Recovery time is less, and it helps me feel more prepared for the next ride. Overall I feel like I put in less effort than I used to. My alignment and stability are stronger, too.

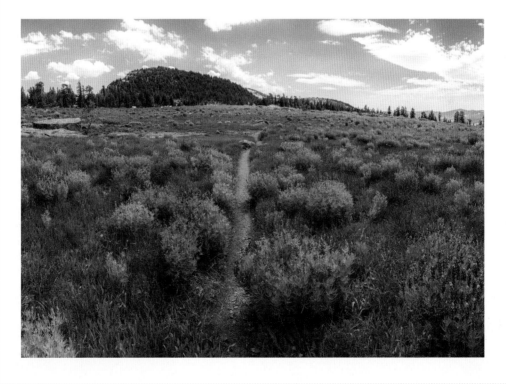

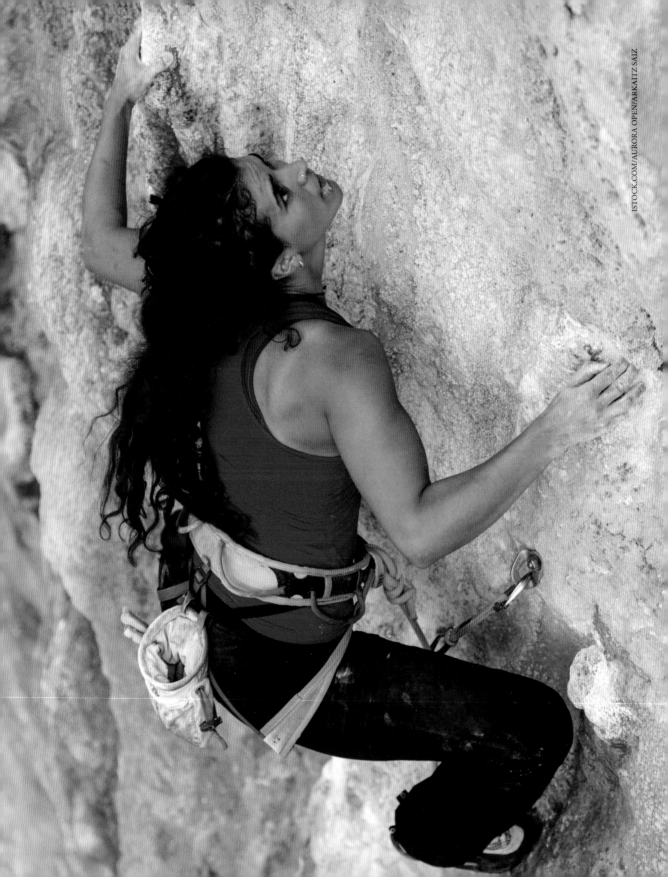

ISTOCK.COM/AURORA OPEN/ARKAITZ SAIZ

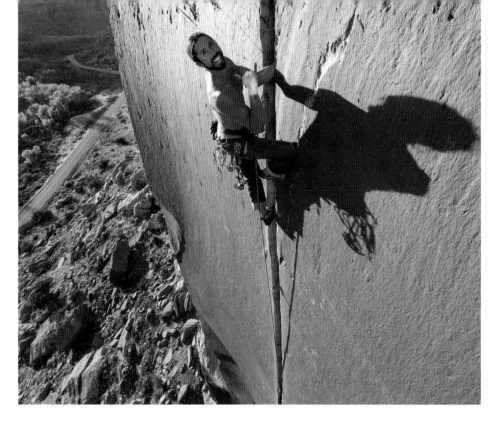

CHAPTER 10

YOGA FOR CLIMBING

In the end, you won't remember the time you spent working in the office or mowing your lawn. Climb that goddamn mountain.
—JACK KEROUAC

WHETHER YOU BOULDER OR CLIMB BIG WALLS, you know the exhilaration of climbing is addictive. It's a demanding sport that pushes all your limits but takes you to some of the most incredible places and experiences. It requires you to be a team player, patient, ever mindful, and endlessly prepared. Hanging on narrow ledges, clinging only to fingerholds, brings you face to face with yourself and nature in pro-found ways. I have so much respect for both indoor and outdoor rock climbers; they are one tough bunch and a tight community that typically stewards the land they climb on and around. If you are an experienced climber or just beginning, incorpo-rating yoga practice into your life will support your climbing on so many levels.

> **YOGA CAN HELP BALANCE FLEXING AND PRONATING WITH EXTENSION AND SUPINATION OF THE FOREARMS AND INCREASE ECCENTRIC MUSCLE STRENGTH."**

Climbing is a demanding sport that takes incredible total body strength, mobility, focus, and practice. It creates mental toughness, deep courage, and problem solving abilities. Obviously the hands, arms, shoulders, core, and legs need to be strong. Hand, wrist, elbow, and shoulder injuries are common for many climbers. Yoga helps relieve the tension and overuse of the arms and hands while increasing overall muscular balance and improving coordination, focus, breath awareness, and recovery.

Meditation and breath practices can help climbers who are facing fears and processing setbacks, injuries, or losses, as well as create a regular space for self-reflection. The incredible demands climbing places on mental stamina and toughness can sometimes overshadow the signals from the body and soul. Regularly meditating and practicing techniques such as *nadi shodhana* help the neurological system and increase self-awareness and compassion while bringing the left and right hemispheres of the brain into greater balance.

ANATOMY OF CLIMBING

Nearly the entire body is engaged at different intensities while climbing. Developing muscle endurance is necessary for the significant static isometric muscle contractions involved in climbing. A few areas do the heavy lifting, with the rest of the body supporting the climb. Let's take a look at the primary areas of the body most in demand for climbing.

Hands/Fingers

Though the legs, core, and shoulders are always at work while climbing, the fingers need to be incredibly nimble and strong. Working on different climbing problems builds this strength and endurance, but most climbers also train the hands and fingers outside of climbing.

Gripping of the fingers is a constant in climbing. It can often lead to fatigue and injuries to the forearms and fingers. The constant grip strength needed means climbers are working on their hand and finger strength in between climbing sessions as well. It is also important to stretch the hands and forearms to keep the muscle tissue healthy. Spreading the fingers during yoga practice is a great balance to climbing. Many hand balancing postures also create a lengthening of the forearms that climbers really benefit from.

YOGI INSIGHT

HEIDI WIRTZ

climber, yogi, philanthropist and owner of Earth Play Retreats; CO.

How did you get into climbing?
I grew up in a very outdoorsy family and we spent lots of time skiing, backpacking, and camping. When I was in college I first got into ice climbing. The beauty and power of the outdoors seen from climbing blew my mind. A group of my friends and I began teaching ourselves to climb, and we just dove in. After I had a bad fall, I found a mentor to teach me a more traditional style of climbing and help me refine my skills. Then I was addicted to climbing.

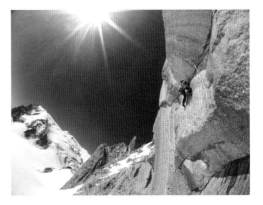

How did you get into yoga?
When I was in college I had really bad sciatica. I bought a book on yoga and started practicing at home. It helped so much. Finally, I found a teacher in the Ashtanga lineage. It cleared my sciatic problem, I had better sleep, and it really helped my climbing. I found that I had better mobility, balance, core strength, and body awareness. Learning about my body, creating breath awareness, and centering my mind became invaluable.

How do you use your yoga practice to support your climbing and guiding life?
I use it before I climb to get centered and calm, warm up my whole body, and increase my focused attention while climbing. After a climb it's so important to unwind. It makes a huge difference when I practice afterwards and speeds up my recovery rate.

How has climbing and yoga changed your life?
I can't imagine my life without both of these activities. I love them. I now lead people on climbing trips, and we always practice yoga. I love the connection to nature and watching people light up, break barriers within themselves and between themselves. Both of these activities draw so many amazing people to our trips.

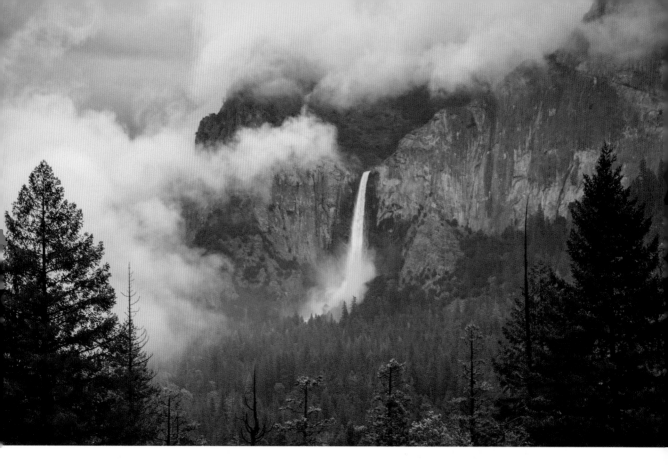

The carpal tunnel of the wrist is a complex and critical component of hand anatomy. The carpal tunnel is a compact area through which finger tendons, blood vessels, and nerves pass from the palm to the wrist, between the carpal bones and flexor retinaculum ligament. Tension in the muscles can press on the nerves in this narrow passage, causing numbness and tingling in the hands as well as tendonitis of the wrist. Practicing yoga can help stretch the muscles that flex the wrist and strengthen its extensors.

Forearms/Elbows

While climbers want to minimize bulk and weight in general (more weight being harder to move), the forearms need to have balanced strength and endurance. The forearm has two compartments: the anterior flexors and the posterior extensors. Straightening and spreading the fingers is controlled by the extensors, while squeezing and making a fist is done with the flexors. There are intrinsic muscles that move the forearm by pronating and supinating the radius and ulna. Extrinsic muscles flex and extend the fingers. The brachioradialis crosses the elbow joint from the upper arm to the wrist and helps extend the elbow joint. Tendonosis is a common repetitive strain injury of the elbow for climbers.

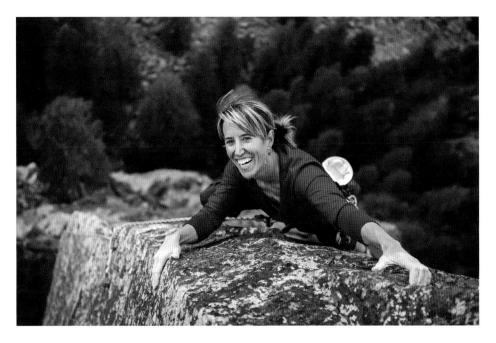

Climbers commonly have strong flexors and weaker extensors, creating imbalances and strain in the wrist, elbow, and sometimes shoulder joints. Training all the different muscles of the forearms and hands is crucial for better holds and endurance. Yoga can help balance flexing and pronating with extension and supination of the forearms and increase eccentric muscle strength.

Shoulders

Imbalances in the shoulders are common for beginning as well as advanced climbers. Sometimes it is due to an injury that didn't heal properly or chronic imbalances that haven't been addressed. The chest muscles (pectoralis major and minor) and latissimus dorsi are often tight, drawing the shoulders and arm bones (humerus) forward, creating strain on the shoulder joint. Rotator cuff injuries, poor posture, and neck strain are common if muscle imbalances persist. Backbending, arm balancing, and inversion postures can help improve posterior shoulder stability, symmetry, and posture.

Low Back/Hips

While not a common site of injury for climbers, low back and hip strain and injuries do happen. If the upper body musculature is imbalanced and overdeveloped, the low back tends to round with the pelvis tucked under. The posterior and anterior hip muscles can be tight and limit healthy movement of the low back and pelvis. Standing postures, sun salutations, backbending, and hip opening postures are all beneficial for balancing the low back and hips for climbers.

Knees

As mentioned in the anatomy chapter, strain and imbalances in the hips often contribute to knee pain and injuries. Additionally, repetitive stress from falling from boulders and walls can damage tendons, ligaments, or the meniscus of the knee joint. Regular moves where the knee is deeply turned in or out create weakness and injury. Edging on small holds or toeing down puts strain on the knees as well.

Backbending, hip opening, standing balancing, and forward folding postures help address imbalances, improve tissue health, and strengthen the knee joint.

Feet/Ankles

Toe injuries, plantar fasciitis of the arch, and ankle injuries are common in the climbing world. Repetitive compression from falls can damage the ankle joints; the arch can become tight and restricted from climbing shoes, toeing, and edging; and the toes are put under immense pressure while climbing. Stretching the feet, ankles, and calves during your barefoot yoga practice helps relieve tension on the joints and create greater balance of mobility and muscle control. All the standing postures of yoga help increase foot and ankle mobility and strength.

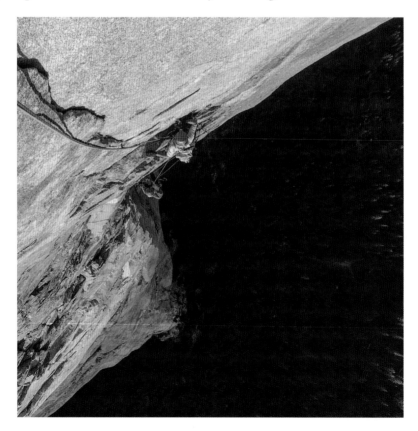

SEQUENCES FOR CLIMBERS

Begin practicing the pre- and post-climbing sequences on your training climbs to prepare your body and improve recovery. Practice the post-climb sequence on your rest days when you aren't climbing to help bring balance to the body and mind. During a multiday climb with limited space, try the short sequence for recovery and preparation for the next climb. Many of these postures can be done either lying down on a mat or sitting in a chair to be more accessible.

Pre-climbing Sequence

Practice this sequence before climbing to prepare the upper body, core, and lower body with the mobility and strength needed to climb.

(1) Joint rotations (see pages 49–51)
(2) Spinal rolls
(3) Cat/cow poses
(4) Downward facing dog pose
(5) Standing forward fold
(6) Sun salutation A (5 sets)
(7) Horse stance with twists
(8) Standing pigeon pose
(9) Locust pose
(10) Reclined twist
(11) Mountain pose

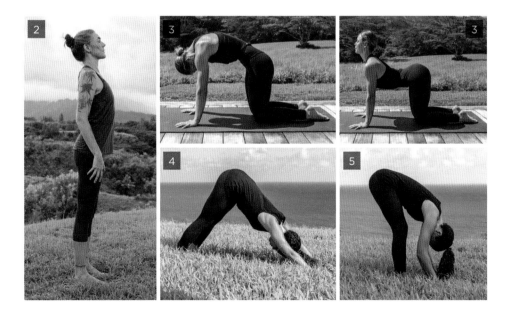

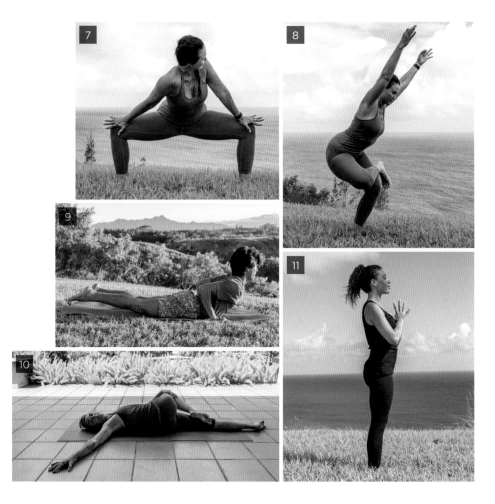

Multiday Climbing Sequence

This sequence is for recovery during a multiday climb. These postures and movements can be done within a portaledge in confined spaces.

(1) Joint rotations, seated and reclined (see pages 49–51)
(2) Easy sitting pose with forward fold
(3) Head to knee pose
(4) Seated forward fold
(5) Reclined twist
(6) Reclined knees to chest pose
(7) Windshield wiper pose
(8) Cobbler's pose
(9) *Nadi shodhana* (10 rounds)
(10) Meditation

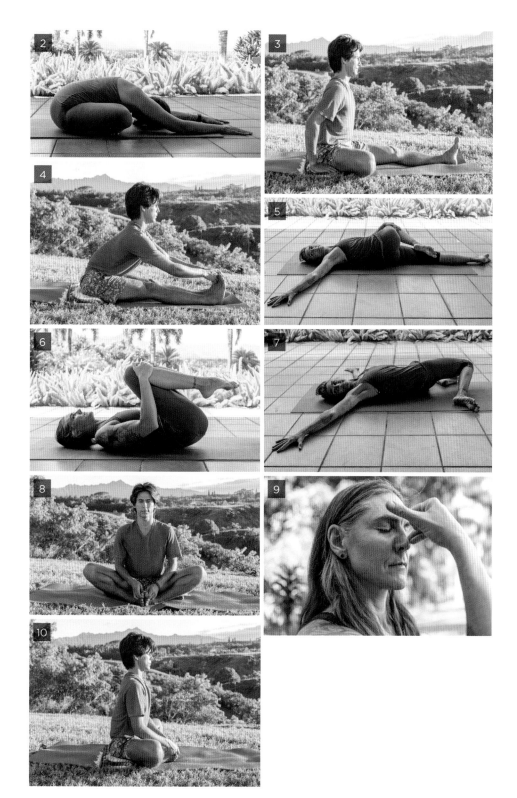

Post-climbing Sequence

To recover after a long day of climbing, try this sequence on solid ground with bare feet and plenty of space and time to unwind from the physical and mental pressures of climbing.

(1) Reclined twist
(2) Reclined hand to big toe pose
(3) Downward facing dog pose
(4) Cobra pose
(5) Child's pose
(6) Bow pose
(7) Puppy pose
(8) Wide legged forward fold
(9) Low lunge pose
(10) Frog pose
(11) Cow faced pose
(12) Seated forward fold
(13) Bridge pose
(14) Plow pose
(15) Corpse pose

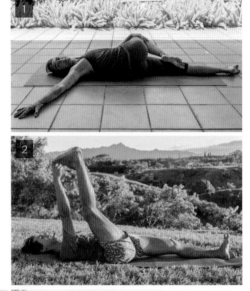

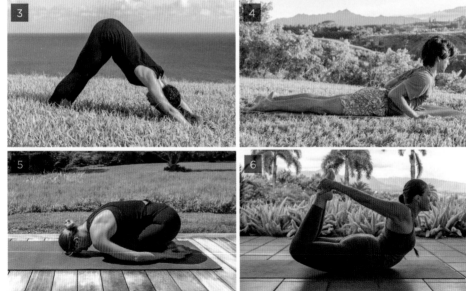

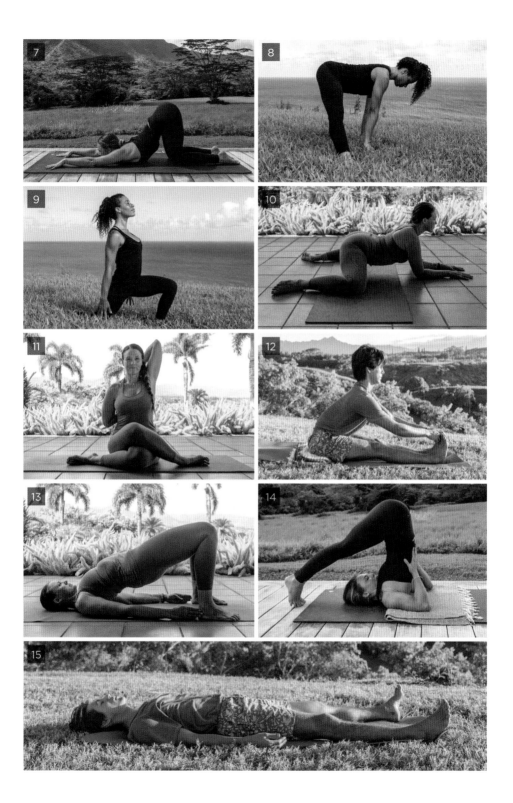

THE TAKEAWAY

Climbing and yoga are such complementary practices. Yoga increases mobility, muscular balance, breath awareness, relaxation response, focus, and full body awareness. Climbing builds strength, focus, presence, and deep respect for life. Many climbers find that having a yoga practice helps them recover faster after climbing and reduces injuries. Whether you are a beginner or an advanced climber, yoga can meet you where you are and help sustain your climbing longer.

- Yoga helps improve musculature balance by strengthening the back of the shoulders, core, and legs.

- Breath awareness improves cardiovascular functioning and endurance.

- Training the relaxation response through yoga practices carries over to climbing sessions.

- Yoga practices help improve overall mind-body awareness, which can help to reduce fear and anxiety during challenges.

YOGI INSIGHT

JOSIE MCKEE

professional climber, NOLS instructor, former Search and Rescue (SAR)
and 200-hour yoga teacher; CA and CO.

How did you get into climbing?
I started climbing indoors at a gym when I was a kid, then got the opportunity to climb outside when I was eleven or twelve. It was terrifying and wonderful! When I was fifteen or sixteen, I went on a climbing road trip to Joshua Tree and was hooked.

What do you love about climbing?
It is such a different and unique way to experience nature and get different perspectives. It teaches me to focus, lead, trust myself, and face fear. The consequences are so real. It's an empowering and mind-blowing experience to be immersed in the wild.

How did you get into yoga?
I started taking classes around climbing, and the more I was exposed to it the more I wanted to practice. My relationship to yoga has evolved alongside climbing.

How has your yoga practice benefited you?
It's so useful to focus my mind, set intentions, and increase my self-control and overall connection to my body. It's improved my mind-body-breath connection on and off the mat. It's helped me through injuries and reducing risk while climbing. I wanted to immerse myself in yoga, so I took a 200-hour yoga teacher training years ago and really got an understanding of the holistic nature of yoga.

How has your yoga practice influenced your climbing?
Climbing is like an *asana* and meditation practice, and I incorporate more and more yoga into my teaching for NOLS. The mental aspect of yoga is so critical in climbing. My yoga practice helps me pay attention when I'm on an edge; it helps me be more aware, calm, and connected. It helps me see what is real and what is not when fears come up. My *asana* practice is a place where I push myself to see past my perceived limitations but also to make wiser decisions as I go, which translates to climbing problems and guiding. I know it makes me a safer climber, too, by minimizing risks and enjoying the experience without attachment to a goal. Practicing yoga after injuries, even visualizing practice, has helped me recover and taught me patience.

What are some mental and emotional benefits you have found through practicing yoga?
The climbing community is tight and the stakes are high. When I have experienced injury or loss, yoga has helped me be okay with my emotions, especially sadness. They are temporary and natural. It's taught me to be more gentle with myself and others. Both climbing and yoga make me a better person, helping me to show up and live better.

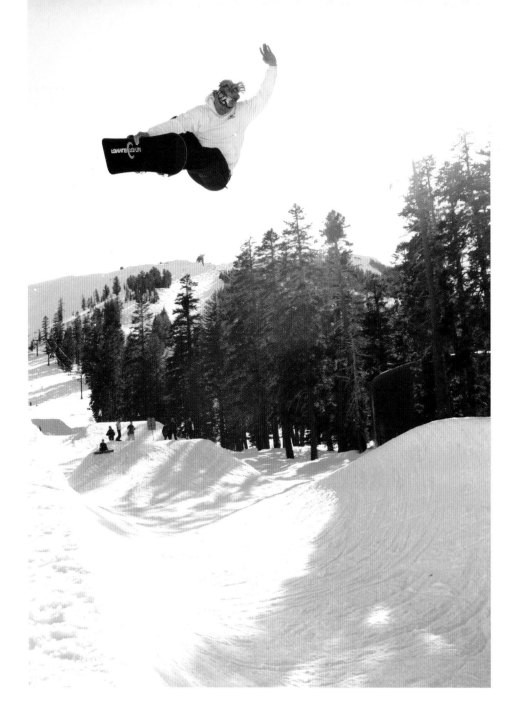

" YOGA HAS BEEN FOUND TO HELP INCREASE BONE DENSITY AND JOINT STABILITY, AND HAS MANY BENEFITS FOR SKIING AND SNOWBOARDING."

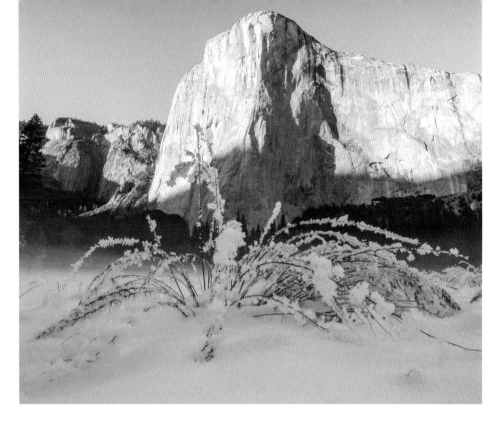

CHAPTER **11**

YOGA FOR SNOW SPORTS

Snow skiing is not fun. It is life, fully lived, life lived in a blaze of reality.
—DOLORES LACHAPELLE

GROWING UP IN FLORIDA, my exposure to snow sports was limited to sledding and snowball fights at my grandparents' home in western Pennsylvania. It wasn't until moving to Michigan during middle school that I had my first taste of skiing. It looked like a ton of fun, but I learned quickly how much hard work it takes to look easy. All snow sports take incredible tenacity to stick with it as you develop strength, balance, and flexibility. Any snowboarder or skier will tell you though, it's all worth it.

Snow sports are full of adventure, fun, and hard work. Patience and dedication build the strength, flexibility, and endurance to crush all day in the mountains at elevation. The scenery can be spectacular, the communities are tight, and the risk factors high. Besides getting out on the mountain, yoga is one of many ways to train and prepare for fun, safe skiing and snowboarding experiences.

Boarding and skiing require skill, strength, mobility, focus, and endurance. Going up and down runs all day uses similar muscles that cycling and running challenge. Temperatures and elevation increase cardiovascular demands. The feet are strapped down, putting the low back and knees at greater risk.

ANATOMY OF SNOW SPORTS

Lower Body

Snow sports of all kinds are very lower body dominant. Ankles need to be strong and flexible in every direction to facilitate movement with the feet strapped down. Deeply bending the knees and stretching the calves in the common skier's stance put extra demand on ankle flexion. The quadriceps muscles of the thighs will be strong and often dominant over the hamstrings, inner thighs, and outer hips. Training your inner thighs and back of the legs, with a mix of strengthening and lengthening, is key to keeping the knees and hips healthy. The high risk of falling or twisting out of a stationary ankle makes knee injuries extremely common in snow sports.

All the standing postures of yoga help to both strengthen and lengthen all the muscles of the legs. Standing balancing poses improve hamstring, inner thigh, and outer hip stability, while the forward folds and wide legged postures improve mobility for the inner thighs and hamstrings. While all the standing postures help improve ankle strength and mobility, low lunges and the seated forward folds and twists create greater flexion—key for all snow sports.

Hips/Core

Skiing and boarding put extra stress on the hips, core, and spine through compression and the increased torque of carving through snow. The muscles of the pelvis need to be both strong and supple for increased range of motion and spinal stability. Because of the need to bend forward slightly at the hips while both boarding and skiing, the hip flexors and psoas tend to be shorter and tighter, which can lead to low back stiffness and pain. Muscles of the back of the hips—the gluteals and lateral rotators—are constantly working and need to be addressed to improve strength and mobility. All the hip opening postures of yoga as well as the standing postures help increase healthy range of motion and flexibility for all sides of the hips. Always

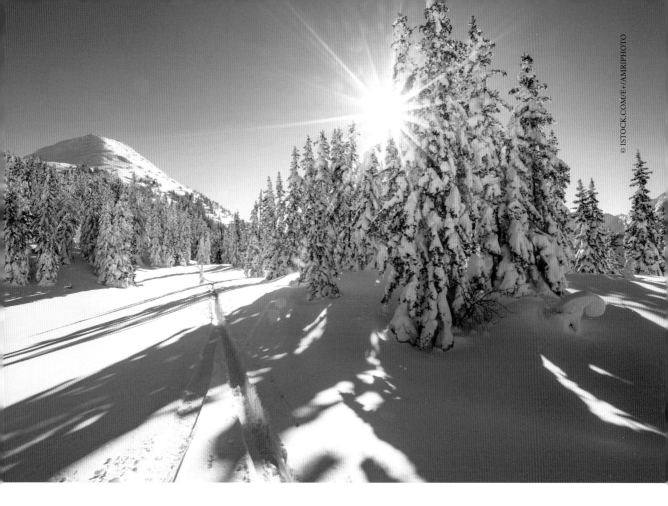

include lunges and some backbends in your practice to open the front of the hips and lengthen the front body.

Core strength is key to support the spine, improve balance, and brace the torso while on the slopes. Plank, hand balancing, and standing balancing postures help create supple and strong core muscles. Incorporate breathing practices into your daily routine for deeper core strength and increased lung capacity.

Upper Body

The upper body is often overlooked in skiing and snowboarding, but is crucial for balance, stability, and turns. Developing your upper body will help reduce the risk of injuries to the shoulders, arms, and back as a result of falling. Broken bones, dislocated shoulders, and muscle strains are common during falls, so everything you can do to increase the strength and mobility of the upper body will help reduce the risks of falling and fall-related injuries. Yoga has been found to help increase bone density and joint stability, and has many benefits for skiing and snowboarding.

Incorporating yoga into your routine can help balance the upper and lower body, and build supple strength and better posture. Sun salutations, arm balancing poses, backbends, and inversions are excellent for building upper body range of motion and stability. Practicing yoga can help build lung capacity and breath awareness as well as improve mental focus and acuity. Add meditation and breathwork to your practices to get the full benefits of the art of yoga.

SEQUENCES FOR BOARDING AND SKIING

Use the pre-slope sequence to warm up and prepare the whole body and begin to practice this sequence on rest days. Practice the post-slope sequence after riding to recover and bring balance to the body and mind. Use the short mid-day sequence as needed to relieve soreness and fatigue. Many of these postures can be done either lying down on a mat or sitting in a chair to be more accessible.

Pre-slope Sequence

This sequence prepares the core, hips, and legs for a day on skis or snowboard. Stay in each posture for five to ten breaths or repeat them a few times each to warm the whole body.

(1) Child's pose
(2) Cat/cow poses
(3) Downward facing dog pose
(4) Standing forward fold
(5) Sun salutation A (5 sets)
(6) Chair pose
(7) Locust pose
(8) Boat pose
(9) Bridge pose
(10) Head to knee pose
(11) Reclined twist
(12) Meditation

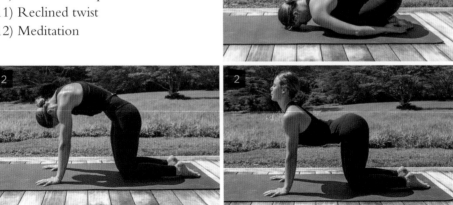

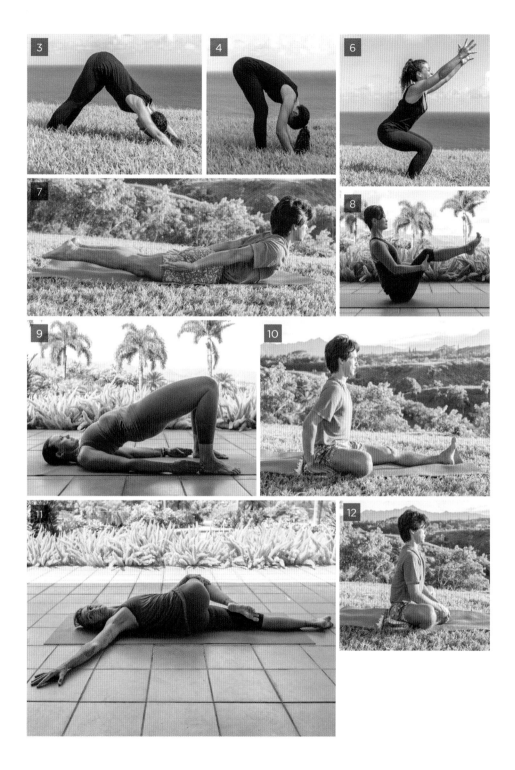

Mid-day Sequence

This short sequence can be done during a break from the slopes to relieve muscle tension and fatigue.

(1) Joint rotations (see pages 49–51)
(2) Upward salute pose
(3) Forward fold
(4) Low lunge pose
(5) Downward facing dog pose
(6) Cobra pose
(7) Child's pose
(8) Simple seated twist
(9) Easy sitting pose with forward fold
(10) Corpse pose

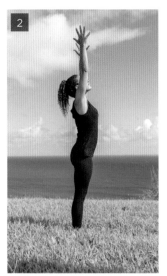

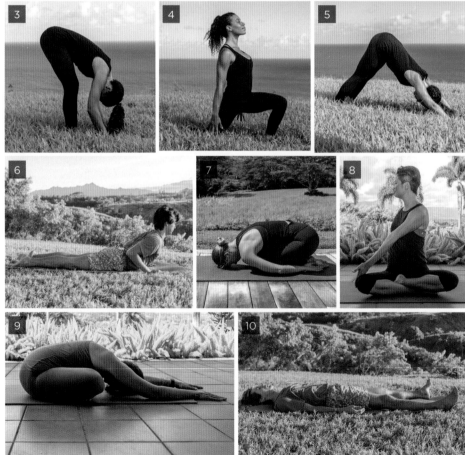

Post-slope Sequence

At the end of a long day, unwind sore muscles with this sequence and recover faster for another day on the slopes tomorrow.

(1) Reclined hand to big toe pose
(2) Windshield wiper pose
(3) Bridge pose
(4) Cat/cow poses
(5) Puppy pose
(6) Downward facing dog pose
(7) Standing forward fold
(8) Cobra pose
(9) Child's pose
(10) One-legged royal pigeon pose
(11) Simple seated twist
(12) Seated wide legged forward fold
(13) Seated hero pose
(14) Reclined hero pose
(15) Happy baby pose
(16) Headstand
(17) Child's pose
(18) Corpse pose
(19) *Nadi shodhana*
(20) Meditation

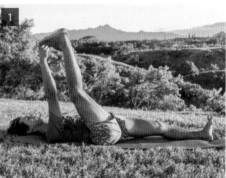

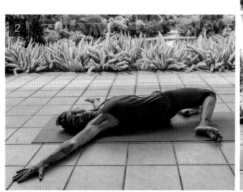

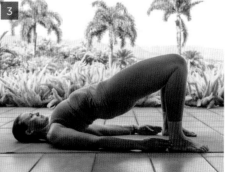

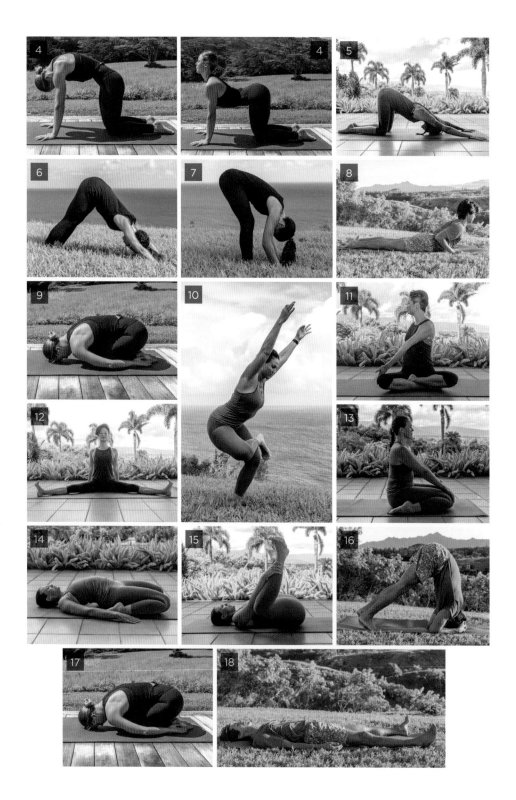

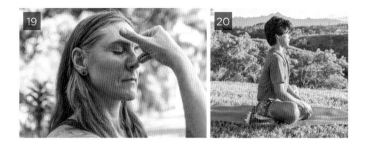

Sequence for Upper Body

It is important to balance the strength of the upper and lower body for skiers and snowboarders. This sequence is great on rest days and for cross-training.

(1) Sun salutation A (5 sets) (aee page 70)
(2) Side angle pose
(3) Triangle pose
(4) High plank pose (hold 30–60 seconds)
(5) Side plank pose
(6) Bow pose
(7) Dolphin pose
(8) Crow pose
(9) Handstand variations
(10) Bridge pose
(11) Wheel pose (3–5 times)
(12) Half lord of the fish pose
(13) Head to knee pose
(14) Headstand
(15) Shoulderstand
(16) Corpse pose
(17) Meditation

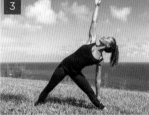

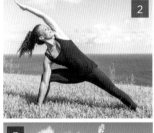

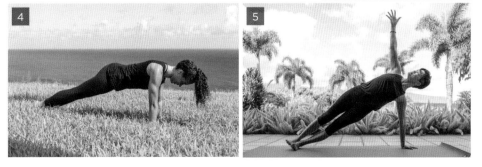

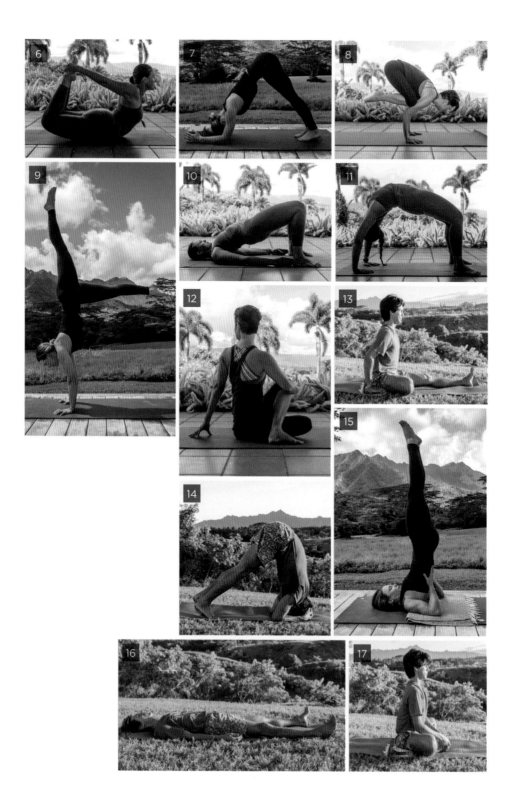

YOGI INSIGHT

BRIDGET PUCHALSKY
licensed acupuncturist, Ayurvedic practitioner, E-RYT 500
yoga instructor, skier and surfer; Santa Cruz, CA.

How long have you been skiing?
I've been skiing since I was a toddler. Growing up in Michigan it was just what we did during the long winters for fun and exercise. It became my social life as a kid and even now as an adult.

How did you get into yoga?
By the time I got to college, after years of skiing my low back started to hurt. There were yoga classes at school so I started going to help with the back pain. Eventually I began to curb my skiing in order to get to yoga class. Yoga was the place I found a philosophy of living and embodiment that I needed.

Besides the exercise, what do you love about skiing?
Being outside, seeing the beauty of nature, plus the powerful cooperative community of the ski culture. It's an ethical thing that skiers understand their connection to nature, the mountains, and have a shared priority to savor life.

How has yoga influenced your skiing?
The eight limbs of yoga help me embody life and live in deeper relationship with nature. I realize that the ancient yogis were mountain people too, living at high altitude at one with the mountains. Yoga is the balance to skiing and other sports. It helps me recover faster, and have less pain and fewer injuries. I have more awareness and connection to my body and can manage my energy better on the slopes.

YOGI INSIGHT

KENNY GRAHAM

E-RYT500 yoga instructor, former pro snowboarder and surfer;
Santa Cruz, CA.

How did you get into snowboarding?
When I moved to Vermont for school everybody was boarding, and I just got into it and was pretty good. All I wanted to do was ride and I started competing.

How has yoga influenced your snowboarding?
I noticed fewer injuries, faster recovery time, and a different mindset. When I injured my knee, I did meditation and visualization practices. I worked on my mental and spiritual strength as I recovered, and when I went back out I tried new tricks I had practiced mentally. As I continued to compete along with practicing yoga, I found that the snowboarding lifestyle just didn't match what I wanted for my future. Yoga supported the lifestyle I wanted.

What do you love about boarding now?
I love the connection to nature and I feel more present when I'm riding. I can feel everything and am in the flow. My relationship with boarding has evolved; I ride with my kids and have so much fun, still.

What's your practice like after riding?
It's slower with longer holds. I begin supine and focus on relaxation, calming, and grounding. I do postures to lengthen my spine and open my hips and chest. Inverting reverses gravity and helps me integrate. Deep breathing practices help me down-regulate my nervous system.

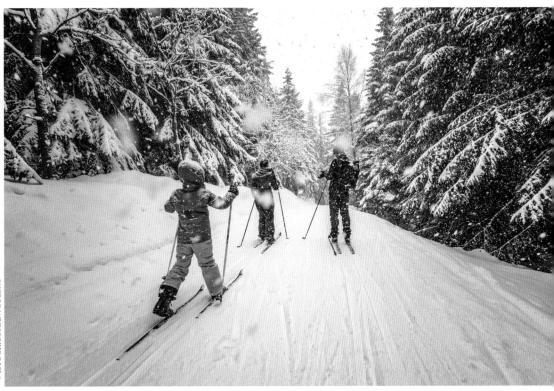

THE TAKEAWAY

Snowboarding and skiing are fun, intense, full body sports promising adventure and great health benefits. Snow sports are dynamic and demanding yang-style practices, while yoga can be a great complementary yin practice. Snow sport enthusiasts can gain a lot of core and upper body strength from practicing yoga daily. By balancing the intensity of time on the slopes with warm up and recovery time on the mat, athletes can create a much more sustainable and enjoyable approach to play time in the powder.

- Skiers benefit from warming up the lower body and core through yoga practice before hitting the slopes.

- A regular yoga practice helps address any misalignments or imbalances in muscles and posture, thereby reducing risk of injury.

- *Pranayama* and meditation can help skiers and snowboarders increase their breath capacity, improve focus and awareness, and gain a deeper sense of calm and centering.

- Practicing yoga after time on the slopes helps in recovery time and improves the post-adrenaline relaxation response.

- Increasing upper body mobility and strength helps improve turns, posture, and balance and reduces risk of injury.

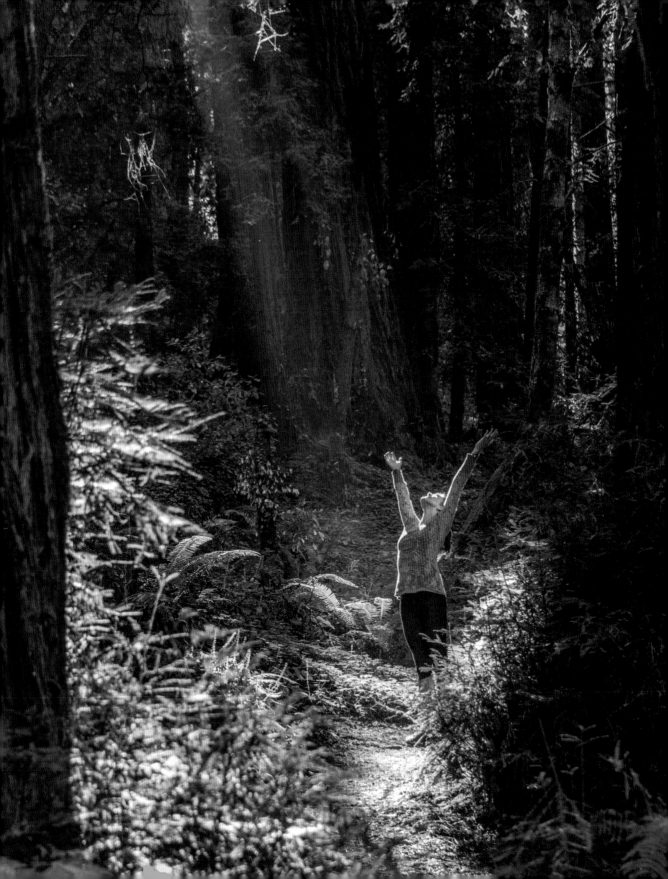

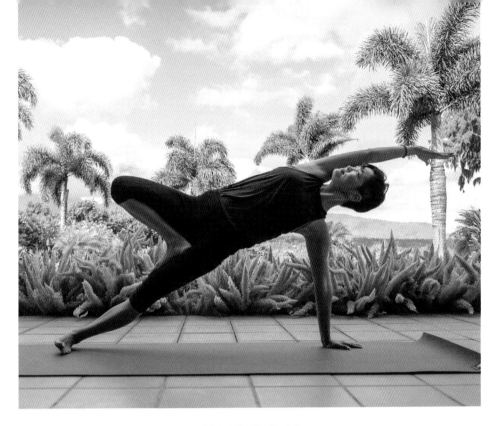

CHAPTER 12

BUILDING A HOME PRACTICE

Yoga is not a work-out; it is a work-in. And this is the point
of spiritual practice, to make us teachable, to open up
our hearts, and focus our awareness so that we can know
what we already know and be who we already are.

—ROLF GATES

IT CAN FEEL OVERWHELMING TO PRACTICE YOGA without the guidance of
a teacher or community of others. Studio classes create a space and time to commit
to the practice, which can be challenging for even the most dedicated athlete to
create on their own, making them an inviting place to start. Whether you are beginning or you have been practicing yoga for a while, it's a good idea to begin a daily

241

> **CREATING DAILY ROUTINES THAT RECONNECT US WITH NATURE AND OUR BIOLOGICAL RHYTHMS HELPS US CREATE A SOLID FOUNDATION FOR HEALTH AND GREATER RESILIENCE TO STRESSFUL TIMES."**

practice. Yoga is an internal practice of awareness and learning about your own body, mind, breath, and spirit. Taking time daily to get deeply connected with yourself on the mat is incredibly empowering. It begins the process of embodying the principles and philosophy of yoga. We develop a deep awareness within ourselves that we can then take into the classroom or out on the mountains, rivers, and boulders.

GETTING STARTED

When I began writing this book, it was still possible to go to a yoga class in a studio, hopefully near your home. Studying with a teacher who is experienced, knowledgeable, and dedicated is one of the best ways to begin practicing yoga. He or she has the ability to see things that you may not see, guide you into appropriate postures, and support you as you struggle, succeed, plateau, and evolve. You also get to meet other people who are also seeking balance, healing, and learning more about themselves through the practices of yoga.

The COVID-19 pandemic changed the yoga studio experience for the duration of 2020, though. Many practitioners suddenly discovered the need for a home practice, and many studios shifted to virtual instruction and various online offerings available to anyone with an internet connection. Whether studios end up reopening or changing entirely, the pandemic changed the yoga class experience in many ways—some that may fade and others that will leave their mark. On-demand classes are incredibly helpful for inspiration and guidance if you are getting started or re-igniting your practice, and have made yoga more accessible to many students. The options can be overwhelming though. In the resource section I have included some online yoga studios that offer a wide variety of classes from some of today's best teachers. Besides that, my goal with this book is for you to have more than enough information to begin your own practice of yoga or get more specific with your practice for your particular needs and sports. Before the internet many of us, myself included, began practicing with a book in front of us. It worked then and still works now.

Practicing in the morning, around the same time every day, helps set up the habit and builds momentum and consistency. You really just need a pleasant, private place big enough for your mat. As your practice deepens and becomes more established, you'll learn to keep your focus while your household carries on around you. One of my teachers practiced in the hallway of his apartment for years, and I had a couple years of practicing in a windowless basement that became my own little sanctuary. If you like to practice outside, find a place with shade and some protection from the elements in order to deepen your focus.

Keep it simple and short. This is key for consistency and learning. A 20-minute yoga practice and 5- to 10-minute meditation every day is more potent over time than an hour once per week. Maybe you get up a little earlier and take some time before you set out for the day, or set aside time after work or before bed. Whatever time of day you choose, try to stick with it for a month, one day at a time. Once your practice is more established, it becomes easier to fit it into your day.

PROPS

All you really need to practice yoga is yourself, some space, time, comfortable clothes to move in, and the intention to practice. Practicing on a hard surface is ideal. Carpet provides extra padding but can make balancing more challenging (which is not necessarily a negative). A yoga mat creates padding and a non-slip surface as well as a sacred space for your practice. When you roll out your mat and get on it, you begin the process of self-care and awareness. There are endless varieties of mats of different lengths, thicknesses, colors, designs, and materials. Do some research and find one that you like, or get an old mat from a friend with some solid practice juju in it (clean it first).

Beyond these tools you may want to get yourself two yoga blocks, a strap, and a blanket. I prefer cork blocks because they are sturdy with a bit of weight. Foam

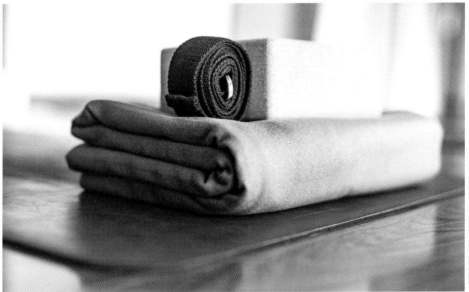

© ISTOCK.COM/ISTOCK/OWNGARDEN

blocks are lightweight and good for traveling. Fancy yoga straps are durable and versatile, but a hand towel, scarf, sarong, or old tie works just as well. Find a blanket that is firm and big enough to fold into a roughly 4-inch thickness. There are so many ways to use folded blankets to support your body in yoga postures and deepen different stretches. Use a blanket under the hips for seated postures if your hamstrings are tight, to make it more comfortable and align the spine upright. Place a blanket under the knees in low lunges or use it under the shoulders for a passive chest stretch.

SEQUENCING

Each of the different sport-specific chapters includes sequences for preparation and recovery. Try different sequences for each sport to help you perform your best. If you are just getting started practicing yoga, begin with the general sequence below that targets every area of the body and the key muscles that are most in need of strengthening and lengthening. Once you get comfortable with practicing daily, begin to explore different sequences based on the ones in the book or classes you have taken. Even experienced practitioners get intimidated with sequencing—it is an art and science unto itself.

General Sequence for All Athletes

Many of these postures can be done either lying down on a mat or sitting in a chair to be more accessible.

(1) Mountain pose (10 breaths)
(2) Joint rotations (see pages __)
(3) Forward bend with knees bent
(4) Sun salutation A (3–5 sets) (see page 70)
(5) Sun salutation B (3–5 sets) (see page 72)
(6) Tree pose
(7) Hand to big toe pose (standing)
(8) Standing pigeon pose
(9) Dancer pose
(10) Warrior two pose
(11) Side angle pose
(12) Triangle pose
(13) Half moon pose
(14) Wide legged forward fold
(15) Warrior one pose
(16) Warrior three pose
(17) Pyramid pose
(18) Revolved hand to big toe pose

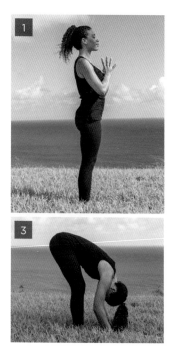

(19) Revolved triangle pose

(20) Locust pose

(21) Bow pose

(22) Bridge pose

(23) Pigeon pose (backbend variation)

(24) Wheel pose

(25) Child's pose

(26) Seated forward fold

(27) Seated wide legged forward fold

(28) Head to knee pose

(29) Half lord of fish pose

(30) *Bharadvajasana*

(31) Fire log pose

(32) Headstand

(33) Shoulderstand

(34) Plow pose

(35) Corpse pose

(36) *Nadi shodhana* (5–10 rounds)

(37) Meditation

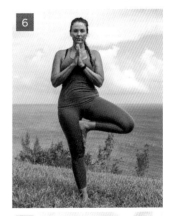

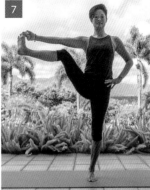

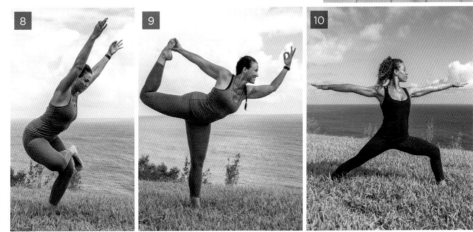

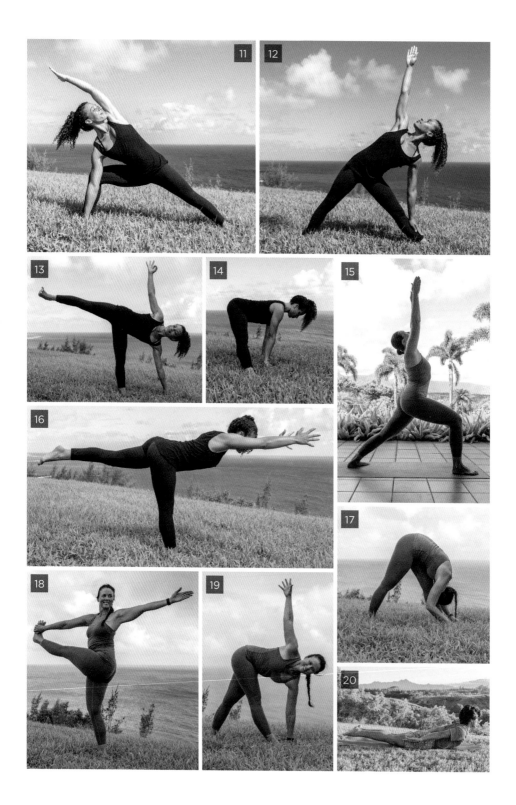

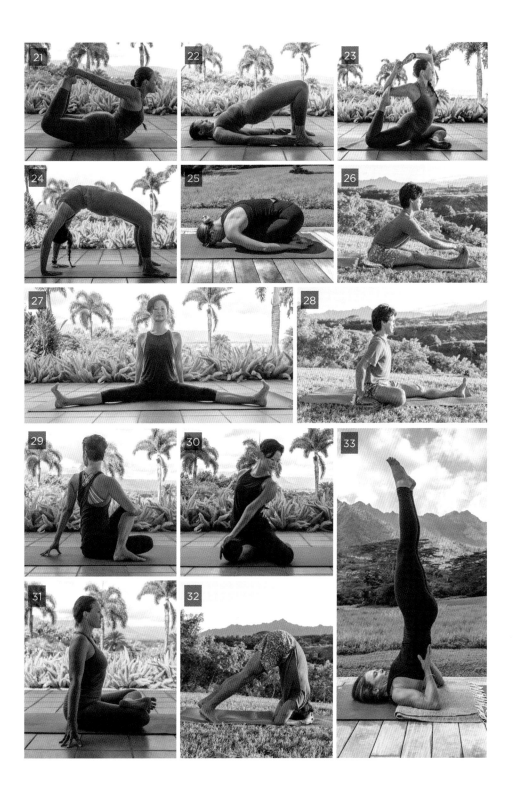

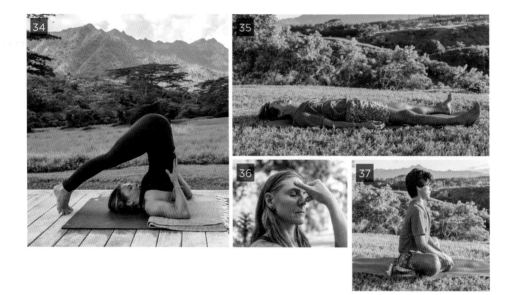

HEALTHY ROUTINES

Practicing yoga, getting regular bodywork, acupuncture, a healthy diet, and sound sleep are all forms of self-care that have incredible benefits when we consciously prioritize them. They are part of daily, weekly, and monthly healthy routines that create a foundation for a super-charged and sustainable life of outdoor adventure for many decades to come.

As humans we have some very basic biological needs that help us find and maintain homeostasis with our environment and changing world. However, modern life has evolved to disregard our circadian rhythms, the cues that our body gives us for sleeping, waking, eating, and working. Our outdoor adventures often have us pushing past these healthy rhythms as we aim to meet our goals. To reestablish our circadian rhythms, we can draw from the ancient science of yoga. Creating daily routines that reconnect us with nature and our biological rhythms helps us create a solid foundation for health and greater resilience to stressful times. Like establishing any healthy habit, it takes time, but once it is part of our routine it supports our overall health. We naturally can rely on these routines to support us through travel, competition, stress, and chaos.

Sleep

Most humans do best with 7 to 8 hours of sleep most nights of the week. Of course there are times when we will get less, but those times will take less of a toll if we are regularly getting enough sleep. Sleep deprivation is so prevalent it has become

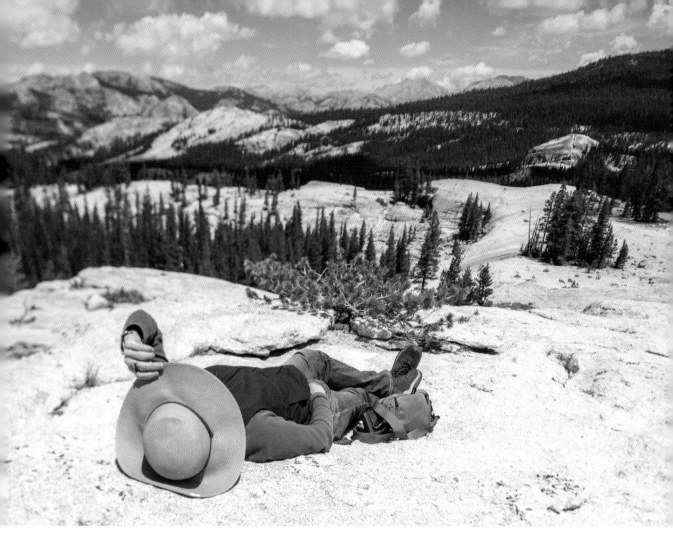

normalized, with one in three adults not getting enough sleep most nights. There is a long list of different issues that arise from chronic lack of sleep, such as blood sugar imbalances, brain fog, loss of coordination, and increased susceptibility to stress. The key is to retrain your body and mind to sleep better and more as much as you can. It all begins earlier in the day. Be sure to reduce your caffeine intake, get exercise daily, reduce screen time at night, and eat at least 2 to 3 hours before bed. As much as possible, aim to be in bed by ten o'clock or so, and try to wake up with the sun unless you are injured, ill, or otherwise exhausted.

Elimination

Healthy elimination is important for so many reasons, and can also be thrown off so easily by travel, diet, poor sleep, and stress. Once you get out of bed, yoga encourages the brushing of teeth, scraping of the coating of the tongue, and elimination of urine and feces. For some this happens naturally, but for others it takes some time and movement to move the bowels. By cleaning the mouth, teeth, and colon, we create a healthy, clear space for the digestive system to work properly throughout the day.

Hydration

Yoga and its sister science of Ayurveda recommend drinking a cup of hot water with lemon in the morning. Ingesting warm water first thing in the morning hydrates the body, stimulates the bowels, and improves the pH of the digestive system. Drink water or herbal tea throughout the day, avoiding iced or cold drinks as much as you can, especially before eating, as it slows digestion of fats considerably.

Movement

As an outdoor athlete you probably don't need more encouragement to exercise, but perhaps consider a different approach. Moving the body during the first part of the day helps increase overall energy, gets your heart rate up, and can elevate your mood for the rest of the day. By exercising, training, or practicing yoga during the cooler part of the day, you also help moderate your energy levels, allowing for a second movement or play time later in the day.

Food

It is beyond the scope of this book to dive into dietary theory, so let's keep it simple here. The philosophy of yoga is to wait until you are hungry to eat, avoid eating a full meal before exercising intensely, and eat fresh, seasonal food that agrees with your system. Aim to have your biggest meal in the middle of the day and a lighter dinner to optimize digestion and assimilation. This creates a stronger digestive system that can be more resilient to changes in routine and diet, especially when you are out on a multiday adventure or training hard.

Play

While training and competing are great, making time for non-competitive play is crucial. It awakens creativity, mental flexibility, and pure joy to feed body, mind, and soul. Later in the day when energy is waning is a beautiful time to let yourself get creative, play, try something new, or get inventive with your yoga practice. Play music, dance, play on a slack line or with your pup—it all helps bring us back to our childlike wonder and happiness and balance out the challenges of sports and life.

Rest

While sleep is crucial, so is simple rest. Letting ourselves slow down, read in a hammock, meander around a lake, fish, dream, write, and gaze at the stars helps us sync up with deep reservoirs of relaxation and wisdom. We so often move from one thing to the next in life, even on a trail, a slope, or river, trying to meet our goals or arrive at a destination. Taking time at the end of the day to simply allow ourselves to listen, observe, and open our senses to the mystery of nature is healing. This is a great time for a restorative yoga practice or meditation as well.

THE TAKEAWAY

One of the most beautiful aspects of yoga is that it is an internal practice that provides the opportunity to know ourselves more deeply and practice on and off the mat. We can practice any time of year, anywhere in the world, and, really, any time of day. Practicing at home can provide you a much needed sanctuary space of healing, right inside your own body, mind, and heart. It is a radical practice of self-care that changes how we engage with others, with our sports, and with nature. As many yogis say, it helps us be better humans in the world and make wiser choices with the gift of our lives.

- Yoga is more a way of living in tune with yourself and the world around you than a set of postures or exercises to perform.

- Essentially you only need yourself and some time to practice yoga.

- Props are extremely beneficial for anyone practicing yoga, as they help us practice movement, breathwork, or meditation with greater alignment and support.

- While you can purchase specific props for yoga, you can also use many items you already have on hand.

- Practicing yoga at home gives you sacred personal time to check on and care for yourself daily.

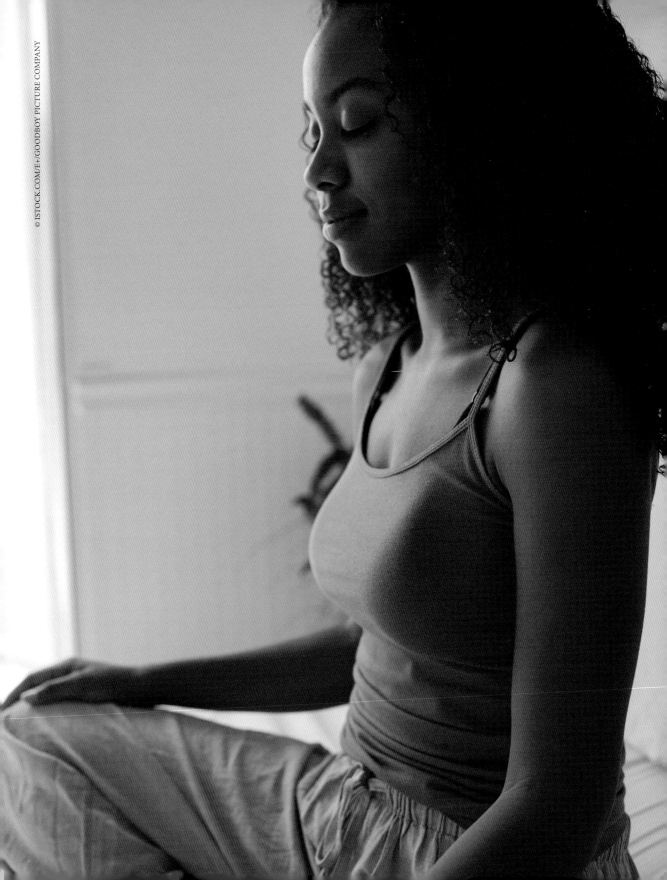

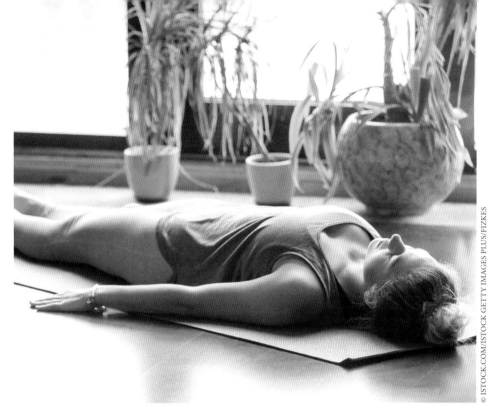

CHAPTER **13**

YOGA FOR RECOVERING

Most of the things we need to be most fully alive never come in busyness. They grow in rest.
—MARK BUCHANAN

GIFTS OF RECOVERY

Every athlete eventually learns the necessity and benefits of recovery time. This is when our muscles actually build, and our body has a chance to integrate training and activity and rejuvenate for the next day or adventure. Overtraining can lead to stress injuries, fatigue, and burnout. By incorporating a regular yoga practice into your life, you are actively recovering through the breathing, moving, attention, intention, and

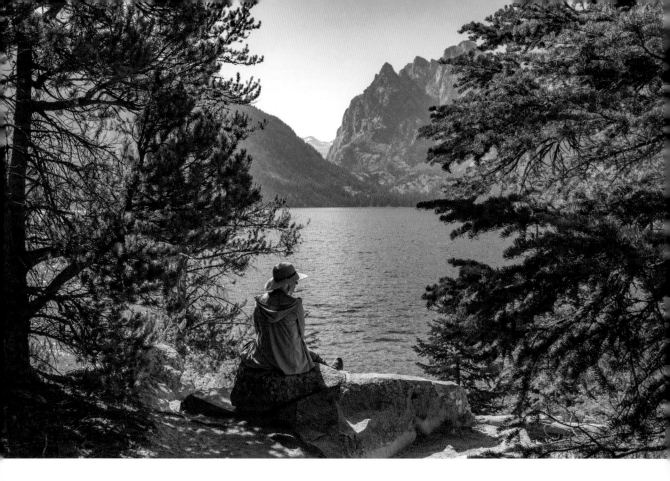

meditative quality it generates. But there is a deeper layer to recovery and healing that can be found in the practice of restorative yoga, meditation, and *yoga nidra*. I suggest building a daily meditation practice and sprinkling restorative postures into your week. *Yoga nidra*, the yogic sleep, is described below and can be added to the end of a practice or done on its own once a week or monthly for a deep reset.

RESTORATIVE YOGA

In my classes I often call this type of practice advanced simply because it is a radical act to consciously slow way down, be fully present with ourselves, and stay in a posture for 5 to 20 minutes without fidgeting. Simply breathing in a posture without moving gives the body, mind, and heart sacred time for releasing stored stress and deeply changing patterns in the nervous system. Restorative yoga is a far more gentle practice than the more athletic forms of yoga that are popular now. The practice is mellow, slow, and uses many props to support the body in different positions to allow a slow relaxation and release response. Studies have shown that restorative yoga improves symptoms of anxiety, depression, stress, and pain as well as improves recovery time after surgery or injury.

Restorative yoga postures are typically simple shapes that are supported with props, as many as necessary, so that we can stay in the pose for a longer period of time and relax deeply. If the posture is uncomfortable at first, add more props until your body and breath can relax. I encourage athletes and type A personalities to do at least one restorative posture at the end of each practice. You can also make a whole practice of restorative postures, which is a wonderful way to rejuvenate your whole being on a rest day.

Because the body cools down during restorative yoga, it is best to have layers on plus an extra blanket to cover the body. If you are in a studio setting you may have access to lots of props, but if you are practicing at home or on the road your props will be limited to what you have on hand. Classic props for restorative postures include two blocks, a strap, one to two folded blankets, and a bolster. When I am on the road or in the backcountry, I use water bottles instead of blocks, my backpack in place of a bolster, and my sleeping bag or a sarong as blankets for support and for warmth. Handkerchiefs or scarves can easily be used in place of a yoga strap. It's helpful to have a timer to use so you don't have to think about how much time you have been in a pose.

SUPPORTED CHILD'S POSE

Begin with your knees wide apart and place a bolster between your legs close to your body. Lengthen your spine forward and lay your chest and head on the bolster with your head turned to one side. Your forearms can rest on either side of the bolster with the shoulders relaxed. You may like to pull a blanket up over your back as you relax. Stay for 5 minutes or so, then turn your head the other direction and stay for another 5 minutes. While in the pose, focus on breathing and relaxing each part of your body.

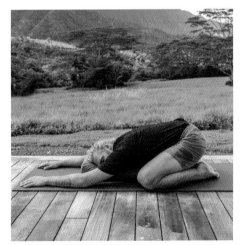

SUPPORTED BRIDGE POSE

This posture is wonderful for opening up the front of the thighs, lengthening the abdominal muscles, and relieving tension in the tops of the shoulders. It's one of my favorites after a day of backpacking. Begin by lying on your back with your knees bent, feet on the ground, and a block next to you. Pressing down into your feet and your arms, lift your pelvis upward high enough to place the block underneath your sacrum at the medium or tallest setting. Let your pelvis rest on the block with your arms at your sides, 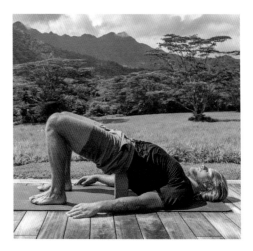 resting for 5 to 10 minutes. Let your head be heavy and the back of the neck lengthen, and focus on your breath as you release your body weight into the block.

SUPPORTED BACKBEND

For this posture you will need a bolster placed across the top half of your mat. Sit in front of the bolster with your knees bent and feet on the ground. Lie back over the bolster until your shoulders are on the ground. You may need to place a blanket under the shoulders for more comfort. Once you release back over the bolster, take five to ten long breaths, relaxing. If it is comfortable for you and does not cause back

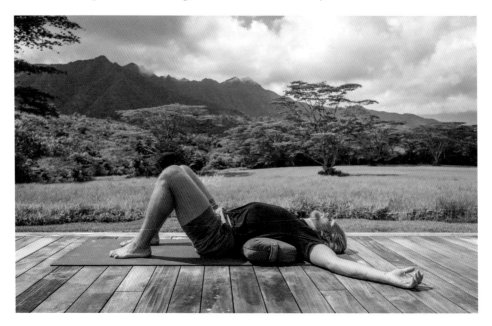

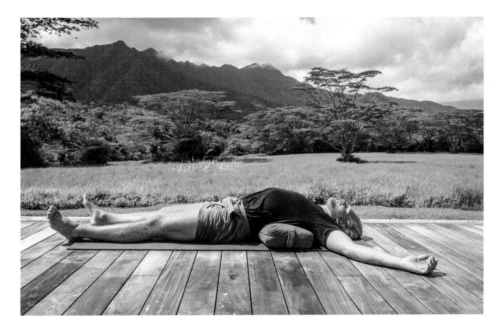

pain, you might extend your legs out long on the mat to lengthen the entire spine. Your arms may be out in a "T" position or extended overhead if that is comfortable on your shoulders. Aim to stay for 5 to 10 minutes in the posture. It is probably the most "intense" of all the restorative postures, so take extra support as needed.

SUPPORTED FORWARD BEND

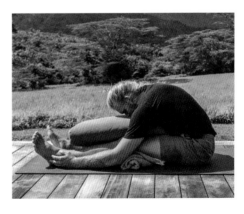

Most of our athletic activities require a strong back and legs. This posture helps lengthen the back of the body and release deeply held tension along the spine. It can be very challenging for the hamstrings, gluteal, and back muscles, so I recommend one bolster and one to two blankets for this pose. Start by sitting on your mat with your legs extended in front of you. If sitting up like this is challenging for you, place a folded blanket under your sit bones. Place a second rolled blanket under the back of your knees to support the legs and ease the tension of the hamstrings. Place the bolster lengthwise on top of your legs and bow forward at the hips, laying your belly and chest on the bolster. Your head may be turned to one side with your hands crossed on the bolster supporting the head, or you may have the forehead down. Stay for 5 to 10 minutes, focusing on long breaths and relaxing the back of your body.

SUPPORTED INVERSION

Reversing the effects of gravity on our bodies is so helpful in relieving fatigue, improving circulation, and reducing swelling in the legs especially. This posture is excellent at the end of every day but especially after long days on your feet. Find a wall or a tree, or use a chair with some clear space in front of it to lie back on. You might also like to have a folded blanket under your head to support the neck. Start by sitting with one hip close to the wall or tree, then gently lower your back down to the ground, extending your legs up the wall or tree. Place the blanket under the head and extend your arms either out to the side or in a "goal post" position. Let your legs relax and get heavy against the support, staying for 10 to 15 minutes. Let your whole body relax, and focus on your breathing as you rest.

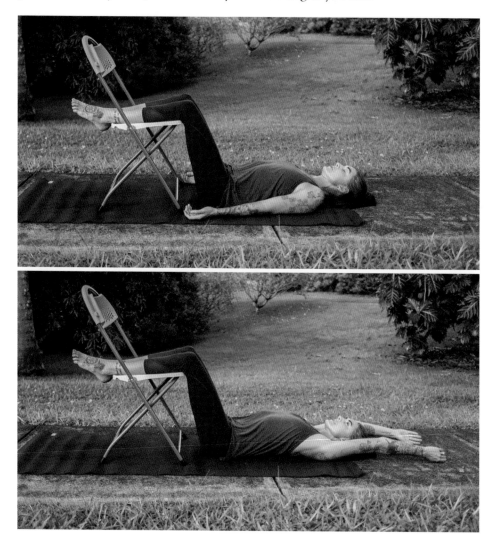

MEDITATION

Dhyana, meditation, is a technique for focusing and stilling the constant fluctuations of the mind. As more space is created between thoughts, we can begin to perceive what lies beneath the surface chatter. Meditation has been practiced for thousands of years as a way of connecting to and understanding the mystical forces within and around us. Today, more and more people are turning to the practice to manage stress. Doctors and therapists are recommending meditation

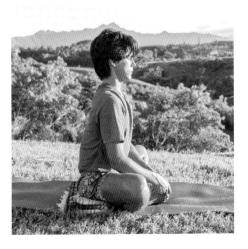

to their patients, and professional athletes of every kind have begun to practice. Reasons to practice differ among students, athletes, and even times of life. I began my own meditation practice decades ago as a way of establishing a home within myself I would always have. Through the years it continues to be a refuge, but the depth of the practice changes depending on the phase of life I am in. Whether you begin to meditate for the mental, emotional, and physical benefits or for the spiritual benefits, meditation will have profound effects on your life.

Breath Meditation

This technique is very simple and yet can generate a profound sense of well-being. Simply focus on the inhalation and exhalation of your breath. As you do you may begin to perceive the nuances during inhaling and exhaling, the different qualities and increasing depth of them. Begin by sitting upright either in a chair or on the ground with a cushion supporting your pelvis. Consciously release tension in your face, neck, and shoulders. Let your hands rest either on your lap or on your knees with a comfortable, soft palm. Take a few moments to connect with yourself and your breath. Then internally repeat the word "in" during your inhalation and the word "out" during your exhalation. Continue breathing and internally repeating the words for 5 to 20 minutes. When your mind wanders away from the breath and the words, kindly bring it back to the breath and begin again.

Notice what sensations and other thoughts arise in your awareness as you do this meditation. There are no wrong thoughts or feelings. When we begin to slow our minds down and connect to the body via the breath, we become aware of all kinds of information. Pain, heaviness, fatigue, calm, joy, sadness, and more lie under the surface of our busy mental activity. Take a few minutes afterward to reflect on the experience and any insight gained.

Body Scan Meditation

Begin by sitting either in a chair with your feet planted and your spine long or on a blanket with your legs crossed. Close your eyes and watch your breath. Just notice how you are breathing, where you feel it, the length and pace. As you watch your breath, it will naturally begin to expand, lengthen, and slow down.

Keeping your breath flowing and natural, begin to slowly scan your body. Notice places of tension or pain. Simply notice at first. Once you have observed any places of resistance in the body, take a few deeper breaths. Let the whole body feel the inhalation and exhalation.

Take your attention to the head. Soften the muscles of your forehead, eyes, mouth, and the back of the skull. Let your tongue get heavy and relaxed. Consciously melt tension from within the head. Then move your attention to your neck and shoulders. Let the tension release as deeply as possible as you breathe. Next take your focus to your right arm, relaxing the muscles and feeling the weight of the arm. Let your fingers soften. Take your focus to your left arm now, feeling into the length and volume of the arm. Let the fingers soften and the palms grow heavy.

Move your attention now to the chest, and let your chest and belly soften as you inhale and exhale. Feel the ribs move, the sternum lift and fall, and the volume of the torso. Next take your focus to your sides. Let them expand and contract with your breath. Just observe and relax deeply. After a few minutes here, move your attention to the back. Feel into the muscles, the structure of the spine, and, once again, the volume of the torso. Take your awareness deeper into the organs of the body. Feel the heart beat.

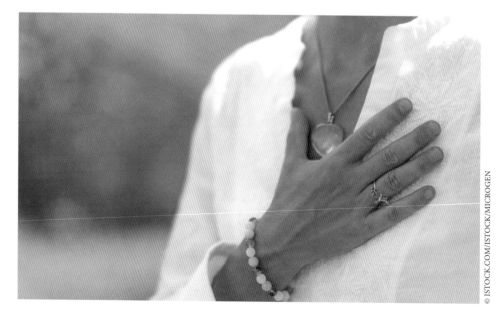

© ISTOCK.COM/ISTOCK/MICROGEN

After you have spent a few minutes just feeling into the torso, move your focus to your hips. Let the breath move into the low belly, and soften any tension in the pelvis as you can. Watch resistance and let the breath flow. After a few minutes here, move your attention to your right leg. Feel the weight, the length, the volume, and any sensations in the right leg. Let your awareness rest here for a bit. Once you feel complete here, move your focus to the left leg. Once again, feel into it from the surface of the skin to deep within the bone.

Lastly, bring your awareness to the whole of your body. Breathe and feel into your body as a whole entity, alive, pulsing, changing, and growing. Let your mind rest inside this awareness of your whole self for as long as you like. When you are ready to bring yourself out of meditation, take a few deeper breaths. Move gently at first and give yourself some time to be slow and gentle before getting into other activities.

Yoga Nidra

Known as the yogic sleep practice, this is an incredibly deep meditation during *savasana*, also known as corpse pose. Anyone can do this practice anywhere. It is a profound healing tool that can be used during illness or injury and can be done any time of day when you can rest without being disturbed for 15 to 30 minutes. There is no right or wrong way to practice *yoga nidra*. You may fall asleep during part of it, forget a section, it doesn't matter. You will still receive the deep relaxing benefits of the practice, which helps us train the deep relaxation response and shift our systems into the healing parasympathetic response. Some of the many benefits are better sleep, faster healing, deeper sense of peace and calm, improved mood, and reduction of physical discomforts.

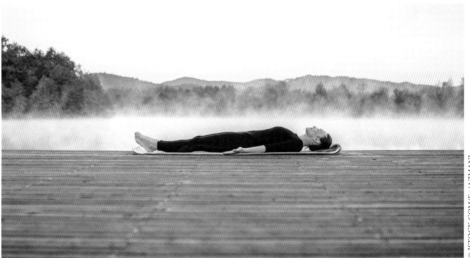

Below is a sample *yoga nidra* script for you to practice. I recommend recording yourself reading the script and using the recording to guide you through the practice until you feel comfortable doing it on your own. Because the body cools down in the practice, wear layers and place a blanket over yourself in corpse pose. Use as many props as you like to feel supported and comfortable.

STAGE 1. PREPARATION

Bring your attention to the space around you. Listen to the sounds outside the room. Listen to the sounds inside the room. Open up your senses: sounds, smells, temperature, feel, and even the taste within your mouth. Visualize your own body resting on the floor, and become aware of your own physical presence. Allow your breath to be natural and easy. Make any adjustments to your posture now.

STAGE 2. MOVING INWARD

Take your awareness inside for a moment and see if you can discover a place of safe haven within. Someplace where you feel at peace, secure, loved, and calm. It can be any part of your body. Let your attention rest there. Spend a moment visualizing this place, and know that you may return to it at any time during this practice, or indeed at any time during your life, when you need it.

STAGE 3. BODY SCAN

Now bring your awareness back to your body resting on the floor. Stay as still as possible, letting your mind rest on each part of the body for just a moment. Notice if any specific parts of your body are more difficult to sense. Sense the entirety of your body all at the same time. Feel your entire being breathing and resting.

Now bring your attention to your breath. Feel the breath entering into the body through your nostrils. Follow the breath as it moves into the chest and abdomen. Then follow the breath as it moves from abdomen to chest and back through the nostrils. Feel enlivened by the inhale and relaxed by the exhale. Sense each breath as energy, and count your breaths up to twelve and then back down again.

STAGE 4. WELCOMING

Without judging or trying to change anything, acknowledge any feelings and emotions that are currently present within you. If you notice something specific, like tension, for example, acknowledge how that feels. Now try to imagine the opposite feeling or emotion by visualizing yourself as happy, healthy, strong, etc. Set an intention for the practice of *yoga nidra*, such as cultivating peace, joy, and courage or releasing control, sadness, or fear. Let this process happen at its own pace.

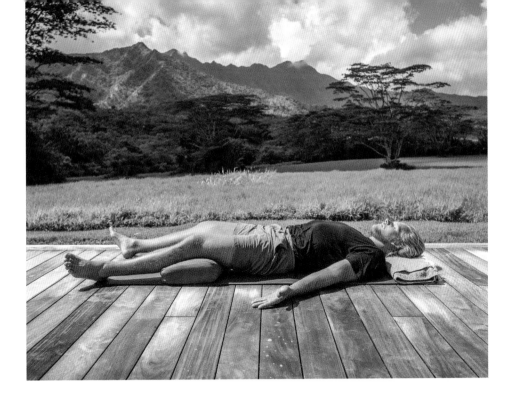

STAGE 5. WITNESSING

Come back to your breath for a moment and notice any thoughts, memories, or images that might arise. Suspend judgment about whatever comes up for you. Now allow images to just float through your mind. A ball. A sky. A home. A field. A flower. An apple. A lake. A shoe. Someone smiling. The sun. A safe place. A good friend. A bird. Someone laughing. A sunset.

STAGE 6. ALLOWING JOY

Bring to mind a memory that holds great joy and peace for you. Then linger here, imagining and remembering all the details of this memory. Let your mind rest here in this happy memory for a little while, generating the feelings in your heart and body.

STAGE 7. REFLECTION

Reflect on how this practice has made you feel. Remember and repeat your original affirmation or intention. Then begin to move outward again, becoming aware of your body and breath. Become aware of the room around you. In your own time, begin to move away from your practice, moving your body, changing positions, stretching slowly. Now the practice of *yoga nidra* is complete.

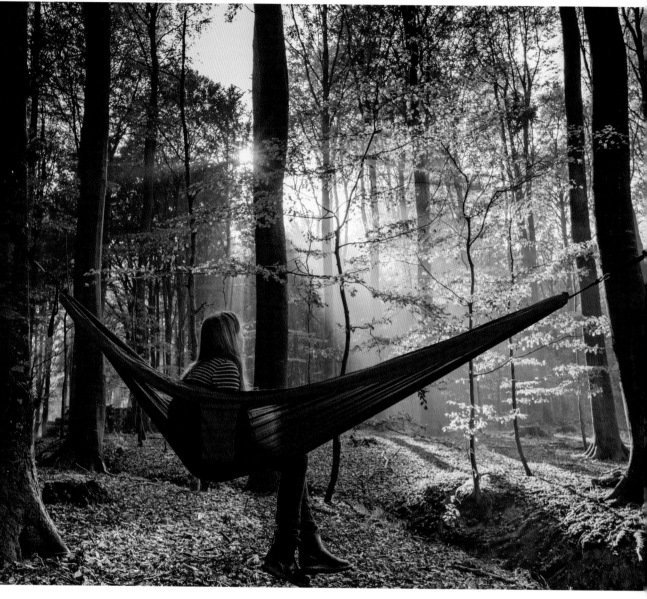

THE TAKEAWAY

There are times to push through and then there are times to rest and recover. Sometimes we have to push through training, competition, barriers, and adventures to meet our goals. Our bodies and minds are often on high with the sympathetic nervous system running the show. If we don't take the time to rest and recover when we can, our systems can get stuck in the "on" position, a place where we are living at a heightened state but not a peaceful one. This not only erodes our physical health and ability to heal but also can start to affect our mental health and emotional resilience. By practicing and incorporating recovery yoga into your routines, you build in rest time and create a stronger foundation of habits to sustain the journey of an adventurous, full life.

- End your regular yoga practice with one or two restorative postures three times a week.

- Aim for one full restorative yoga practice weekly and especially after hard training, competition, or an adventure.

- Start to build a daily meditation practice. Begin with 10 minutes. Once that is a habit, lengthen the time of sitting. Use the body scan meditation as a guide or tap into one of the meditation sources listed in the Resources section of this book.

- Record the *yoga nidra* practice for yourself or have a friend record it if you like. Then use the recording to guide yourself through the practice once a week, perhaps at the end of a restorative practice.

- Most restorative postures as well as meditation and *yoga nidra* are excellent practices while you are injured or ill to maintain and improve your ability to heal and integrate changes.

- These practices are highly recommended for improving sleep, mood, peacefulness, and a positive mindset.

REFERENCES

Bouanchaud, Bernard. *The Essence of Yoga: Reflections on the Yoga Sutras of Patanjali.* Portland, OR: Rudra Press, 1997.

Calais-Germain, Blandine. *Anatomy of Movement.* Seattle: Eastland Press, 1993.

Center for Outdoor Ethics. "The 7 Principles." Leave No Trace, https://lnt.org/why/7-principles.

Clark, Sara. "An Introduction to Restorative Yoga." *Very Well Fit*, January 14, 2020.

Kapit, Wynn, and Lawrence M. Elson. *The Anatomy Coloring Book*, 4th ed. New York: Pearson, 2013.

Keil, David. *Functional Anatomy of Yoga.* West Sussex, UK: Lotus Publishing, 2014.

Kempton, Sally. *The Heart of Meditation.* South Fallsburg, NY: Siddha Yoga Publications, 2002.

Kerouac, Jack. *The Dharma Bums.* New York: Penguin Books, 1971.

Lasater, Judith Hanson. "Seeking Samadhi." *Yoga Journal*, April 5, 2017.

Laskowski, Edward R., MD. "What Are the Risks of Sitting Too Much?" Mayo Clinic, May 8, 2018. https://www.mayoclinic.org/healthy-lifestyle/adult-health/expert-answers/sitting/faq-20058005?utm_source=facebook&utm_medium=sm&utm_content=post&utm_campaign=mayoclinic&geo=national&placementsite=enterprise&mc_id=us&cauid=100502&linkId=98336428.

Levesque, Anna. *Yoga for Paddling.* Guilford, CT: FalconGuides, 2017.

Lipton, Bruce, PhD. *The Biology of Belief: Unleashing the Power of Consciousness, Matter & Miracles*, 10th anniversary ed. Carlsbad, CA: Hay House, 2016.

Mayo Clinic. "Walking: Trim Your Waistline, Improve Your Health." Healthy Lifestyle: Fitness, February 27, 2019. https://www.mayoclinic.org/healthy-lifestyle/fitness/in-depth/walking/art-20046261.

McGonigal, Kelly, PhD. *Yoga for Pain Relief: Simple Practices to Calm Your Mind and Heal your Chronic Pain.* Oakland, CA: New Harbinger Publications, 2009.

Muir, John. *Our National Parks.* New York: Gibbs Smith, 2018.

O'Rahilly, Ronan, Fabiola Müller, Stanley Carpenter, and Rand Swenson. "Basic Human Anatomy: A Regional Study of Human Structure." Dartmouth Medical School, 2004. https://www.dartmouth.edu/~humananatomy.

Schultz, R. Louis, PhD, and Rosemary Feitis, DO. *The Endless Web: Fascial Anatomy and Physical Reality.* Berkeley, CA: North Atlantic Books, 1996.

Stephens, Mark. *Teaching Yoga: Essential Foundations and Techniques*. Berkeley, CA: North Atlantic Books, 2010.

Swanson, Ann. *The Science of Yoga: Understanding Anatomy and Physiology to Perfect your Practice*. New York: DK, Penguin Random House, 2019.

RESOURCES

Adaptive Yoga Live: This is a fantastic resource for learning adaptive yoga postures and practices for yourself and loved ones. www.adaptiveyogalive.com

Balanced Rock Foundation: This is a nonprofit organization that leads community yoga classes in the Yosemite National Park area and summer retreats focused on yoga, hiking, writing, and connection to nature. www.balancedrock.org

Breathe Together Yoga: My former yoga home in San Jose, California, this studio has fantastic and highly trained teachers, online classes accessible to all, and workshops and trainings. www.breathetogehteryoga.com

David Kiel: David and his website are a wealth of current anatomy information and training. www.yoganatomy.com

Earth Play Retreats: This is the organization Heidi Wirtz formed to teach people climbing and yoga. www.earthplayretreats.com

Elemental Yoga: This yoga training and classes are based in functional movement science and classical yoga. www.elementalyogatraining.com

FalconGuides: An incredible resource for all things outdoors, from sports to wildflowers, wildlife, and camp cooking. www.falcon.com

Functional Range Conditioning (FRC): Functional anatomy seminars are a great place to dive deeper into functional movement training for any sport. www.functionalanatomyseminars.com

Leave No Trace: This site is full of information and training on Leave No Trace principles and practices. Before you go out into nature, give it a thorough read please. www.lnt.org

Mind Body Paddle: Anna Levesque's home for all things paddling, yoga, and Ayurveda, including retreats, consultations, and classes. www.mindbodypaddle.com

Mindful: This is a wonderful resource for mindfulness and meditation training and practice. www.mindful.org

Mobility IQ: This training system combines yoga, functional range exercises, breathwork, and meditation to increase body awareness, strength, and mobility. www.mobility-iq.com

NOLS: The National Outdoor Leadership School is based in Lander, Wyoming, but hosts outdoor adventure courses around the world. They are the home of Wilderness First Responder (WFR) trainings, which are held at different locations around the United States and beyond. www.nols.edu

US National Park Service: Before you adventure into any park, check out the latest information about the park, weather, permitting, restrictions, and accessibility. www.nps.gov

Yoga International: This is a fantastic and high-integrity resource for all things yoga and meditation. There are many excellent teachers, articles, and trainings to choose from. www.yogainternational.com

INDEX

A

abdominals, 21, 24
active recovery pose, 52
adductors, 20
adho mukha svanasana, 58
agni stambhasana, 124
ananda balasana, 132
anjaneyasana, 67
ankle, 19, 51, 218, 228
arches, 147
ardha bekhasana, 97
ardha chandra chapasana, 79
ardha chandrasana, 79
ardha hanumanasana, 126
ardha matseyandrasana, 108
ardha pincha mayurasana, 134
arms, 172
asana, 5
ashta chandrasana, 67

B

backbends, 95
backpacking, 167
badha konasana, 128
bakasana, 94
bharadvajasana, 109
bhujangasana, 61
biceps brachii, 23
biceps femoris, 20
bicycles, 93
bipedalism, 144
bitilisana, 56

blisters, 152
boat pose, 91
body scan meditation, 260
bound angle pose, 128
bow pose, 98
brachioradialis, 23
breath, 41
breath meditation, 259
bridge pose, 99
bridge press, 54
bunions, 152

C

camel pose, 100
candlestick pose, 135
cat pose, 56
chair, 48
chair pose, 66
chaturanga dandasana, 59
child's pose, 55
clavicle, 22
cobbler's pose, 128
cobra pose, 61
connective tissue, 17
contraction, 17
core, 89, 154, 172, 228
corpse pose, 261
cow faced pose, 122
cow pose, 56
crescent lunge, 67
crow pose, 94
cycling, 197

D

dancer pose, 86

dandasana, 119

deltoid, 23

dhanurasana, 98

dharana, 7

dhyana, 7

diaphragm, 24

dolphin pose, 134

downward facing dog, 58

E

easy side-bending pose, 111

easy sitting pose, 116

eka pada rajakapotasana, 103

elbow, 23

elimination, 249

erector spinae, 21

eversion, 19

extended side angle pose, 73

F

fascia, 17

feet, 19, 30, 169, 184, 199, 218

femur, 20

fingers, 214

fire hydrant pose, 57

fire log pose, 124

food, 250

foot, 147

forearms, 216

forward fold, 66

forward folding postures, 126

four limbed staff pose, 59

frog pose, 119

G

garland pose, 120

gastrocnemius, 19

gate pose, 113

gemellus, 21

gluteal, 21

goddess pose, 87

gomukhasana, 122

gracilis, 20

H

halasana, 139

half frog pose, 97

half lord of the fish pose, 108

half moon pose, 79

hamstrings, 20

hand, 36, 216

handstand, 136

hand to big toe pose, 83

hanumanasana, 121

happy baby pose, 132

headstand, 140

head to knee pose, 127

heel spurs, 152

hero pose, 101

high plank, 59

hindolasana, 123

hip, 21, 50, 153, 171, 184, 217, 228

hip opening postures, 115

horse stance, 87

hovering table, 89

humerus, 22

hydration, 250

I

iliacus, 21

iliopsoas, 21

intercostals, 24

inversion, 19

inversions, 133

isometric, 17

J

janu sirsasana, 127

jatthara parvattasana, 110
joint rotations, 49

K
knee, 19, 31, 51, 152, 218, 228

L
latissimus dorsi, 21
leaping monkey pose, 121
leg lifts, 92
legs, 170, 184, 199
levator scapulae, 22
lizard lunge, 117
locust pose, 60, 96
low back, 171, 217
low lunge pose, 67

M
malasana, 120
mandukasana, 119
marichyasana, 107
marjaryasana, 56
meditation, 259
mindfulness, 9
mountain pose, 63
multifidi, 21
musculoskeletal system, 17

N
nadi shodhana, 43
natarajasana, 86
navasana, 91
neck, 37, 49, 172
niyamas, 4
    ishvarapranidhana, 4
    santosha, 4
    saucha, 4
    svadhyaya, 4
    tapas, 4

O
oblique, 21
obturator externus, 21
obturator internus, 21
one-legged royal pigeon pose, 104

P
paddling, 182
padmasana, 125
parasympathetic response, 43
parighasana, 113
parivritta hasta padangusthasana, 85
parivritta sukhasana, 106
parivritta trikonasana, 81
parivritta upa vistha konasana, 114
parivritta utthan pristhasana, 118
parsvottanasana, 80
paschimottanasana, 129
pectineus, 20
pectoralis, 21
pelvis, 32
peroneal, 19
piriformis, 21
plantar fasciitis, 151
play, 250
plow pose, 139
pranayama, 6, 42
prasarita padottanasana, 77
prasarita balasana, 112
pratyahara, 6
pronation, 23
pronator teres, 23
props, 243
protraction, 22
psoas major, 21
puppy pose, 58
pyramid pose, 80

Q
quadratus femoris, 21

quadratus lumborum, 21
quadriceps, 20

R
radius, 23
reclined centering, 52
reclined full extension, 55
reclined hand to big toe pose, 131
reclined knees to chest pose, 52
reclined twist, 54
recovery, 253
rectus abdominis, 21
rectus femoris, 20
respiratory system, 24
rest, 251
restorative, 254
retraction, 22
reverse warrior, 75
revolved hand to big toe pose, 85
revolved triangle pose, 81
rhomboids, 21, 22
rotator cuff, 22
royal pigeon pose, 103
runner's stretch, 126

S
salamba sarvangasana, 138
salamba sirsasana, 140
samadhi, 7
samshitthi, 63
Sanskrit, 48
sartorius, 20
savasana, 261
scapula, 22
seated baby cradle, 123
seated forward fold, 129
seated staff pose, 119
seated wide legged forward fold, 130
semimembranosus, 20
semitendinosus, 20

sequencing, 244
serratus anterior, 21, 22
setu bandha sarvangasana, 99
shalabhasana, 96
shoulder, 22, 35, 49, 172, 217
shoulderstand, 138
side-bending child's pose, 112
side-bending postures, 111
side-bending wide legged pose, 114
side plank , 90
simple seated twist, 106
skandasana, 88
skiing, 227
sleep, 248
snowboard, 227
soleus, 19
spinal extension, 95
spinal rolls, 51
spine, 18
standing crescent pose, 65
standing forward fold pose, 66
standing pigeon pose, 84
sternocleidomastoid, 23
sternum, 22
subscapularis, 22
sukhasana, 116
sun salutations, 70
supination, 23
supine twist, 110
supported backbend, 256
supported bridge pose, 256
supported child's pose, 255
supported forward bend, 257
supported inversion, 258
supraspinatus, 22
supta padangusthasana, 131
supta virasana, 101
surya namaskar, 70, 72
sympathetic nervous response, 43

T

table twists, 57
tada kapotasana, 84
tadasana, 63
tensor fascia latae, 21
teres minor, 22
tibialis anterior, 19
toe stretching pose, 102
torso, 21, 154, 185
transverse abdominis, 21
trapezius, 21, 22
tree pose, 82
triangle pose, 78
triceps brachii, 23
twisted thigh stretch, 118
twisting postures, 106

U

ujayii, 43
ulna, 23
upavistha konasana, 130
upward facing dog pose, 62
upward facing wheel pose, 105
upward salute pose, 64
urdhva dhanurasana, 105
urdhva hastasana, 64
urdhva mukha svanasana, 62
urdhva mukha virkshasana, 136
ustrasana, 100
utkatakonasana, 87
utkatasana, 66
uttanasana, 66
utthan pristhasana, 117
utthita hasta padangusthasana, 83
utthita parsvakonasana, 73
utthita trikonasana, 78

V

vasisthasana, 90
vastus intermedius, 20
vastus lateralis, 20
vastus medialis, 20
viparitha karani, 135
viparitta virabhadrasana two, 75
virabhadrasana one, 69
virabhadrasana three, 76
virabhadrasana two, 74
vrksasana, 82

W

walking, 144
warm up, 48
warrior one pose, 69
warrior three pose, 76
warrior two pose, 74
wheel pose. *See* upward facing wheel
    pose
wide legged forward fold, 77
wind relieving pose, 53
windshield wiper pose, 53
wrist, 50, 216

Y

yamas, 3
    ahimsa, 3
    aparigraha, 3
    asteya, 3
    brahmacharya, 3
    satya, 3
yoga nidra, 261

ABOUT THE AUTHOR

JANA KILGORE is an avid hiker and leads backpacking retreats in Yosemite National Park with Balanced Rock Foundation. She is a 500 E-RYT (500-hour Experienced Registered Yoga Teacher) with the Yoga Alliance and a board-certified Ayurvedic practitioner through NAMA, a clinical nutritionist, herbalist, chef, and licensed massage therapist. She is part of the lead faculty for WildYoga YTT (yoga teacher training) and teaches public classes through Breathe Together Yoga. She currently lives on Kauai, Hawaii, with her partner, photographer/chef/waterman Patrick Bremser and their dog, Faith.

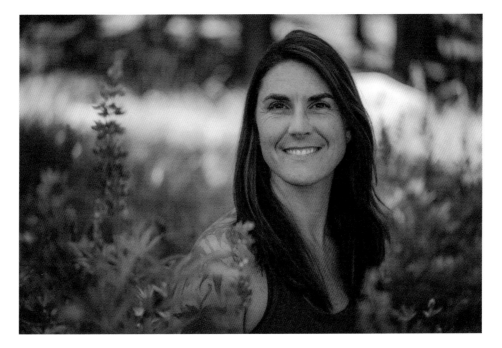

ABOUT THE CONTRIBUTORS

QUINN BRETT is a lifelong outdoor athlete and accomplished big-wall climber, yogi, and advocate for public lands. After a life-altering fall in 2017, she now continues her advocacy, athletics, and accessibility work from her wheelchair. She works for the National Park Service expanding and improving the accessibility programs in all the parks, writes, and continues her yoga practice. She is a courageous force for change and an incredible human being.

PATRICK BREMSER is a culinary artist, photographer, woodworker, and a lifelong waterman. He is a classically trained chef who cooks for private clients and is always crafting delicious experiments. When he's not in the kitchen, he's either working with wood or in the ocean capturing the might and magic of earth, water, and light. He lives on the north shore of Kauai with his wife, author Jana Kilgore, and their pup.